A World Otherwise

A World Otherwise

Environmental Praxis in Minamata

Yuki Miyamoto

LEXINGTON BOOKS
Lanham • Boulder • New York • London

Published by Lexington Books
An imprint of The Rowman & Littlefield Publishing Group, Inc.
4501 Forbes Boulevard, Suite 200, Lanham, Maryland 20706
www.rowman.com

6 Tinworth Street, London SE11 5AL, United Kingdom

British Library Cataloguing in Publication Information Available

Library of Congress Control Number: 2020946830
ISBN 978-1-7936-4360-5 (cloth : alk. paper)
ISBN 978-1-7936-4361-2 (electronic)

Contents

Acknowledgments

While I was revising this manuscript, *A World Otherwise*, I came across a book that carries a similar title, *Otherwise Worlds*: *Against Settler Colonialism and Anti-Blackness*.[1] Although the anthology *Otherwise Worlds* focuses on racial inequality and the discourse of colonization, which my manuscript does not directly discuss, both books explore the possibilities of and seek for a way to realize a world that is operated differently than this modern world. Thus, I am pleased by the prospect that a world otherwise may not be too abstract but is already incubating and flourishing like this anthology. I hope that this book, *A World Otherwise*, will foster an imagination for an alternative world in readers' minds.

This *world otherwise* that I examine is the one envisioned by Minamata sufferers and their supporters, particularly Hongan no kai, and will detail the Minamata disease, its history, and Hongan no kai in the following pages. In the meantime, what I discovered from reading books, articles, and Hongan no kai's newsletters, *Tamashii utsure* (Transferring the spirit), was that their religious sensibilities are indispensable in conceptualizing their world otherwise. Although I was unable to examine in this volume Ishimure Michiko's notion of *modae gami*, a deity in agony, or Chisso president Shimada Ken'ichi's Buddhism and his wife's Catholicism, I would like to return to these themes sometime.

In completing this book, I am indebted to the guidance and friendship of individuals and the generous support of institutions and organizations. Discussing the environmental disaster and the economic and social structures of the modern world with my students at DePaul University helps me to think further about the concept of otherwise. Dr Norma Field, Professor Emerita at the University of Chicago, allowed me to accompany her to her trips to Japan, where she kindly introduced me to people in Fukushima and the evacuees from Fukushima after 2011's nuclear accident. These trips gave me invaluable experiences in not only seeing the similarities between Minamata and Fukushima but also witnessing the injustice, inconsistent, and irrational policies that have caused the ongoing plight of the people.

My colleagues in my department—especially Drs. Khaled Keshk, Chris Mount, and Chernoh Sesey—are all encouraging and supportive, which made my journey possible and enabled me to complete this book. In particular, the conversations with Dr. Kalyani Menon inspired me intellectually on numerous occasions and encouraged me countless of times whenever I lost my confidence to finish the project. I am grateful for her intelligence, kindness, and a great sense of humor. A course team-taught at DePaul with Dr. Nobuko Chikamatsu in the department of modern languages was a joy, offering me opportunities to analyze the environmental disaster from a linguistic perspective.

The funding from DePaul University's Quality of Instruction Council (2013–2014) and the Wicklander Fellowship (2014–2016), as well as my paid leave of absence (2017), Association for Asian Studies' Short-term Research Travel to Japan by the Northeast Asia Council (NEAC) (2018) enabled me to travel to Minamata throughout the years. During these trips, Mr Kasai Nobuo of Sōshisha was an invaluable interlocutor. My gratitude also extends to my families in the United States and Japan, who are always on my side and never lost faith in me when I was overwhelmed by the amount of work I faced. Finally, this book will not have come into being without Kanazashi Junpei-san and Hiroko-san. I greatly appreciate their friendship and vision of life.

NOTE

1. Tiffany Lethabo King, Janell Navarro, and Andrea Smith, eds., *Otherwise Worlds: Against Settler Colonialism and Anti-Blackness* (Durham, NC: Duke University Press, 2020).

Introduction

In March 2011, while driving on the busy streets of Chicago, listening to NPR, a piece of news captured my attention: the Fukushima Daiichi nuclear power plant had lost its electricity, urgently necessitating that the cooling system be brought back online immediately to avoid nuclear meltdown. I was still recovering from news of the damage wrought by the massive earthquake and tsunami on the northern coast of Japan, which had taken thousands of lives just a couple of days earlier. The additional news about the malfunctioning nuclear reactors was greatly disturbing. Within a week, three reactors exploded successively. Upon learning about the explosions, I immediately had the impulse to send iodine pills to Japan, in the hope of helping to protect people from thyroid cancer caused by leaking radiation. I made some phone calls, and one of my former students introduced me to his neighbor, a medical doctor who might have access to iodine pills. It did not work out. I called a politician's office in Japan to see whether there was enough iodine on hand, but they were in the midst of a chaotic situation and were understandably preoccupied with helping evacuees and providing immediate care. I had to face my helplessness a thousand miles away from the disaster.

Even after the initial shock and confusion subsided, the situation did not appear any better. Tokyo Electric Power Company (hereafter TEPCO), the utility company which owns the Fukushima nuclear power plant, concealed or distorted certain facts pertaining to the incident (e.g., the company denied the meltdown for five months);[1] the Japanese government withheld important information from the public (e.g., the current of the radiation plume);[2] and the medical community downplayed the significance of radiation exposure (e.g., a medical doctor stated that "the effects of radiation do not come to people who are happy and laughing. They come to people [who] are weak-spirited, [who] brood and fret").[3] TEPCO, the municipal governments in Fukushima prefecture, the central government, and some scientists and medical professionals appeared to me to have withheld crucial information regarding health concerns in the affected areas when the hot spots and the patches of high-level radiation were found within and beyond Fukushima.

After Fukushima's triple disaster of the earthquake, tsunami, and nuclear meltdown, recollections of the aftermath of the bombings of Hiroshima and Nagasaki reverberated, corresponding to growing anxieties and concerns about radiation. Literature, documentaries, news programs and the like treating the matter of radiation exposure became increasingly available: Some materials raised awareness of the danger of living in an environment of low-dose radiation, while others offered instruction for how to cope with it. Some drew upon the cases of Hiroshima and Nagasaki in formulating safety measures; others looked to Chernobyl for models for how to respond to the aftermath. Movie theaters and local communities organized film screenings on the effects of radiation exposure in past incidents, while new films were being made about people in Fukushima.[4] My video library was soon filled with documentaries and dramas about March 11, 2011, and I accumulated articles in newspapers, magazines, and journals that discussed the nuclear accident. In the meantime, I witnessed that words such as *alpha*, *beta*, and *gamma rays*, *cesium*, *half-life*, *external and internal exposure to radiation*, *decommissioning*, and so on entered the everyday vocabulary of people in Japan.

It was not just the events causing radiation exposure that were brought to people's minds. The aftermath of the explosion evoked déjà vu in the people who knew about or were involved in cases of *kōgai*, a term literally meaning *public harm*, but indicating environmental disaster specifically. The uncanny structural similarities between those *kōgai* cases and the ongoing Fukushima incident were striking. For example, author Ishimure Michiko wrote about one notorious case of *kōgai* known as "Minamata disease"—methylmercury poisoning caused by contaminated water released into the Shiranui Sea by the Chisso Corporation for over thirty years, until 1968.

Ishimure's words, though written four years before the Fukushima nuclear accident, conspicuously resonate with the problem surrounding the treatment of the contaminated water from the Fukushima Daiichi nuclear power plant:

> If I remember correctly, the Chisso factory's newsletter once said that the contaminated water would quickly be diluted in the water of Minamata Bay [of the Shiranui Sea]. Japanese modernization breeds an attitude that allows humans to release poison into the water. Given the [Japanese] tradition of worshipping the water deity and venerating the god of the well, I wonder when and how such disrespect [toward the environment and the deity] came into being.[5]

While the earthquake and tsunami that hit the northern part of Japan were extraordinary in their scale, response to the aftermath of Fukushima was, unfortunately, by no means new. Indeed, it was quite familiar for the ways the corporation addressed (or dismissed) its wrongdoing, how governments and jurisdictions treated (or ignored) people's sufferings, and how some medical doctors were complicit with the denials issued by governments and corporations.

The quote from Ishimure continues as follows: "In prioritizing industrialization, contemporary Japanese society has come far from the thoughts expressed in Sugimoto Eiko's advocacy of prayer and Ogata Masato's 'Chisso within' (*Chisso wa watashi datta*). The situation appears incurable."[6] I was, in particular, intrigued by those individuals—Sugimoto Eiko, Ogata Masato, Ishimure Michiko—and I wanted to understand what Sugimoto's forgiveness and notion of *nosari* or gift consisted of, what Ogata's "Chisso within" and *shōgoku* or a birthlace meant, and Ishimure's *furusato* or home in her mythopoetic prose conveys. I wished to learn more both about and from them, whose comments on traditional religion and modern industrialization in Japan suggested that their thoughts might offer resources for considering environmental catastrophe in the context of contemporary ethics. I soon found that these individuals had formed a group called *Hongan no kai* (Association of the Original Vow). Although many individuals and organizations—all of whom would merit attention—have provided various forms of care to those suffering from methylmercury poisoning,[7] in this book, I focus on Hongon no kai, whose distinct religious sensibility offers a model for the practice of countering the "modern" attitude—the attitude that, as Ishimure suggest, has given rise to conditions leading to environmental disaster.

Focusing on the thoughts and actions of the founding members of Hongan no kai, this book attempts to articulate the group's vision of a world in which relationships between humans, their environment, and each other are conceived differently from those that prevail in the modern, industrialized world. Hongon no kai's vision calls for a paradigmatic shift—an ontology reconceived in a manner that recalls Emmanuel Levinas's masterpiece *Otherwise Than Being*. Much as Levinas pursues a new way of construing the self in relation to others while critiquing traditional Western ontology as "egology,"[8] Hongan no kai's members seek to realize a world in which humans define themselves through relationships, not only with other human beings but also with nonhumans and other-than-humans.[9] Echoing Levinas, I refer to Hongon no kai's vision as "a world otherwise."

Considering the specificity and import of this vision, this book examines the praxis—the thoughts and actions—of this group, discerning and articulating their vision of a world otherwise. Toward this end, I examine the group's newsletter and other publications as my primary texts. Drawing upon my disciplinary training in textual hermeneutics to interpret these materials, I situate the group's thoughts and actions explicitly within an environmental ethics framework. Issues of the Hongan no kai newsletter *Tamashii utsure* ("Transferring the spirit") are not readily available at commercial bookstores, but are printed in Japan and available through subscription or by direct purchase at the Hongan no kai office. The small size and limited circulation of the newsletter afford it a sense of trust and intimacy; members of the group are able to share thoughts and news in a frank and relatively uncensored manner. For this reason, examining the newsletter's seventy-five issues will offer special insight into the group's collective sensibility and ideas. Employing my hermeneutical approach, I attempt to discern and make salient the ethical significance of the voices, ideas, and actions of Hongon no kai's members, emphasizing their contributions to the current discourse of environmental ethics. As we will see, Hongon no kai challenges prevailing ontology (concepts of "being"), epistemology (theories and formations of "knowledge"), and ethics (one's relationships with oneself and others), proffering a vision that resists the "modern" attitude that has led to disaster.

I was fortunate to meet Kanazashi Junpei, the secretary of Hongan no kai, who informed me about the group's newsletters. Fascinated by their content, I returned repeatedly to Junpei-san and his wife, Hiroko-san, both of whom welcomed me with open arms when I was still a stranger, just one of many visitors to Minamata. But in conversations with them that often lasted for hours over a course of days, I was drawn to their enchanting stories and way of life, which allowed me to glimpse a world otherwise. The Kanazashis grow cotton, vegetables, and fruit, but do not seek to dominate their natural environment around them. Rather, they struggle with nature—bugs that eat cotton sprouts, wild boars that dig up the roots of the vegetables in the farm, and birds that pick fruit—and even complain about the harshness of natural world. But at the same time, they appreciate its blessings; a mutuality obtains between nature and those who depend on it for food and livelihood. Consequently, the Kanazashis' relationship with their surroundings, which appeared equal and equipotent, enabled me to appreciate the agency of nonhumans and other-than-humans.

My friendship with the Kanazashis challenges romantic views of nature, as well as approaches that see nature in terms of mere commodity. In addition, my encounter with the Kanazashis further fortified my conviction as a scholar that in engaging matters of environmental catastrophe and other tragedies, the field of ethics does well to integrate the voices, thoughts, and actions of the people who have experienced those events firsthand. As postcolonial theory, feminist theory, and critical race theory emerge in response to lived sufferings, so should environmental ethics incorporate the voices of those who experience and contend with environmental catastrophe and degradation firsthand.

In accord with my methodology, the first chapter of this book introduces the notion of *janaka shaba*—or *mou hitotsu no konyo*, the latter of which has conventionally been translated as "another world within this world." The phrase *janaka shaba* circulates widely among the sufferers of Minamata disease and their supporters who yearn for a world in which humans build relationships with nonhumans and other-than-humans differently, and thus conceptualize themselves differently. As I have indicated, I wish to translate *janaka shaba* as "a world otherwise." Not only is "a world otherwise" a more precise translation (a very literal translation would render the phrase "a world not in this way"); it also emphasizes the ontological *difference* that Hongon no kai's vision seeks to realize. Introducing the key facets of this book—Minamata disease, Hongan no kai, and their contribution to environmental ethics—chapter 1 prepares readers for a journey to Minamata.

Chapter 2 unfolds the history of Chisso—the company responsible for discharging water contaminated with methylmercury into the Shiranui Sea—in the context of Japan's modernization process, including its colonization of neighboring countries. Here I locate Chisso not only geographically but also historically and politically in accounting for the role of the corporation in the minds of the Minamata people. In doing so, I consider the meaning of "modernity" in Japan as a system and corresponding set of values.

With this understanding of modernity in place, I turn in chapter 3 to individual Hongan no kai members. Here I relate the life stories of the Sugimotos and their way of coming to terms with Minamata disease and the harassment and discrimination by fellow Minamata citizens they suffered as a result of their affliction. Despite the hardships borne by the entire Sugimoto family, both Sugimoto Eiko and her father Susumu eventually made the decision to forgive Chisso. Like many others, I initially believed that "forgiving" Chisso let the perpetrators off the hook far too easily; the Sugimotos' forgiveness felt unsatisfying and indeed unsettling to me. But as I discuss in this chapter, political scientist Jane Bennett's notion of the "agency of assemblages" proves helpful, if not entirely agreeable, for understanding why and how the Sugimotos arrived at forgiveness. This stance is reflected in the mission statement issued at the inauguration of Hongan no kai, which states, "The Minamata disease incident manifests how terribly our modern industrialized society is suffering. We must not forget that underneath the incident is our own sin and arrogance, which led us to the destruction of our environment and the invaluable lives of people."[10]

Chapter 4 introduces the charismatic and enigmatic figure of Ogata Masato—a fisher, Minamata sufferer (i.e., one who suffers from Minamata disease), activist, and founding member of Hongan no kai. Drawing upon the work of philosopher Giorgio Agamben, this chapter looks to Ogata in order to discuss the possibility of a post-Minamata ethics. After a brief incarceration in a detention facility in Kumamoto city for juvenile delinquency, Ogata returned to Minamata and was actively involved with the first of several lawsuits against Chisso filed on behalf of Minamata sufferers. However, before the final verdict was issued, he withdrew from the lawsuit. As a consumer of the commodities produced by Chisso, Ogata believed himself to be as guilty for the disease-causing pollution as Chisso. Admitting that he thereby enabled the modern system that gave rise to the disease, Ogata provokes questions about the very notion of "agency" in the modern world. As we will see, his insights on this matter constitute an important contribution to environmental ethics, limning the ontology of a world otherwise.

How to realize Ogata's vision is one motivating question for the following two chapters, which treat the life and work of prolific Minamata writer Ishimure Michiko. Chapter 5 focuses on Ishimure's foundational period, prior to her international recognition as a writer. Ishimure's childhood and her experiences as an adolescent shaped her voice as a writer. Ishimure's literature—her novels, poetry, and plays—convey the Minamata people's sufferings. As my interpretation of her work reveals in this chapter, Ishimure's writings deal in what I refer to as the power of the fragile, an element that emerges from Ishimure's encounters with Minamata sufferers and her involvement with one of the Minamata lawsuits.

The sixth chapter investigates Ishimure's "mythopoetic" writing and its indebtedness to the plot of a Mugen Noh play—a genre of Japanese theater. I read this writing as a kind of guide for realizing a world otherwise. Mugen Noh plays are distinct for containing a story within a story; a story narrated by a Buddhist monk encompasses a story narrated by an other-than-human—a ghost, demon, or some other entity that, though not part of "this" world, interacts with this world. Ishimure's work, taking cues from Mugen Noh plays, similarly includes stories narrated by other-than-humans. I argue that Ishiumure's mythopoetic, multivocal prose challenges the "rationality" subscribed to in the modern, monological system that has led to human suffering and environmental disaster on an unprecedented scale. In concluding the two chapters on Ishimure, I analyze the Japanese government's nostalgic rhetoric of *furusato,* or home/land, as part of its campaign to persuade Fukushima residents to stay or return to their "homes." I argue that Ishimure's use of *furusato*, free of the nostalgia of the government's use of the term, functions as a critical counter to this national rhetoric.

The final chapter examines the concrete actions of Hongan no kai. In particular, I focus upon the group's inaugural and ongoing practice of carving stone statues and placing them on the reclaimed land of Minamata. To convey the ideas underpinning this action, I discuss the Japanese context of Jizō bodhisattva, after which many of Hongan no kai's statues are modeled. This figure embodies a rich religious sensibility that extends beyond Buddhism as traditionally conceived. Hongan no kai carve these statues as a way of translating their plights and prayers into tangible objects for all to contemplate, thus inviting others to experience a world otherwise.

Throughout the book, I follow Livia Monnet, the translator of Ishimure Michiko's *Kugai jōdo: Waga minamatabyō* (The Paradise in the Sea of Sorrow: Our Minamata Disease), in referring to people who were affected by methylmercury in Minamata as "sufferers" instead of the "victims" (*giseisha*) or "patients" (*kanja*).[11] I do so because the labels of "victims" and "patients" were used by the Japanese government to determine who was eligible for compensation money. Those who were considered eligible for compensation were commonly referred to as "certified patients" (*nintei kanja*). But as this book in its totality seeks to convey, the sufferings of the people of Minamata must not be reduced to, or by, such bureaucratic nomenclature, which derives from the modern impulse to "compensate" with money that for which money alone cannot compensate.[12] This study of the ethical praxis of Hongan no kai's members challenges such reductions of suffering across many registers, and in doing suggests ways of realizing a world otherwise.

NOTES

1. Jake Adelstein and David McNeill, "Meltdown: What Really Happened at Fukushima?" *The Atlantic*, July 2, 2011. https://www.theatlantic.com/international/archive/2011/07/meltdown-what-really-happened-fukushima/352434/

2. Norimitsu Onishi and Martin Fackler, "Japan Held Nuclear Data, Leaving Evacuees in Peril," *The New York Times*, August 8, 2011. https://www.nytimes.com/2011/08/09/world/asia/09japan.html

3. Yamashita Shun'ichi's statement is found in "Japan Admits 3 Nuclear Meltdowns, More Radiation Leaked into Sea; U.S. Nuclear Waste Poses Deadly Risks," *Democracy Now*, June 10, 2011 https://www.democracynow.org/2011/6/10/as_japan_nuclear_crisis_worsens_citizen and Gayle Greene, "Science with a Skew: The Nuclear Power Industry after Chernobyl and Fukushima," *The Asia-Pacific Journal* 10, no. 1 (3) (2011). https://apjjf.org/2012/10/1/Gayle-Greene/3672/article.html

4. I especially learned from, and was motivated by, Kamanaka Hitomi's series of documentaries. She made her first documentary film (about radiation exposure), *Hibakusha: At the End of the World*, in 2003. The film was inspired by her encounter with a girl in Iraq who had leukemia, due most likely to exposure to radiation from depleted uranium—the radioactive weaponry made of nuclear waste that was used in the Iraq war. She then made *Rokkasho Rhapsody* in 2006, illustrating the everyday lives of people living in Rokkasho mura (village) in Aomori Prefecture, home to a nuclear facility that enriches uranium, temporarily stores spent nuclear fuel, and produces mixed oxide fuel. While she was showing her 2010 film *From Ashes to*

Honey (which explores alternatives to nuclear power, focusing on the residents of the small island of Iwaijima and their attempts to resist the construction of a nuclear power plant across the sea, comparing their efforts to those in Sweden) at a theater in Shibuya, the earthquake interrupted the film screening on March 11, 2011.

5. Ishimure, Michiko, *"Minamata Mandala wakai hōkoku 'Mirai e no teigen' Katariau dai ni bu 'Minamata ga jinrui ni hasshite irumono'"* ("The Minamata mandala report on reconciliation 'Suggestions from the future, part two, The message from Minamata to humankind'"), *Tamashii utsure* 29 (2007): 27–28.

6. Ishimure, *"Minamata Mandala wakai hōkoku,"* 27–28.

7. For example, Sōshisha, Gaia Minamata, and Hotto Hausu helped Minamata sufferers. Especially, Hotto Hausu, established by Katō Takeko, accommodates the Minamata sufferers who were exposed to methyl mercury in utero.

8. Emmanuel Levinas, *Totality and Infinity: An Essay on Exteriority*, trans. by Alphonso Lingis (Pittsburgh, PA: Duquesne University Press, 1969), 44.

9. The term "other-than-humans" is coined with Frédérique Apffel-Marglin in her book, *Subversive Spiritualities: How Rituals Enact the World* (New York: Oxford University Press, 2011). More explanations will be given in chapter 1.

10. Hongan no kai newsletter, *Tamashii utsure* (Transferring the spirit), no. 1 (1998). The English translation was the original. In *Tamashii utsure*, no. 6 (2001), page 5, they call themselves the "Club of the Original Vow," but I will use their Japanese name, *Hongan no kai*, throughout this book.

11. The following sentences from Susan Sontag are suggestive to think of the nature of suffering: "Etymologically, patient means sufferers. It is not suffering as such that is most deeply feared but suffering that degrades. That illness can be not only an epic of suffering but also the occasion of some kind of self-transcendence is affirmed by sentimental literature and, more convincingly, by case histories offered by doctor-writers." Susan Sontag, *Illness as Metaphor and AIDS and Its Metaphor* (New York: Picador, 1988), 125.

12. To recognize as a "certified patient" (*nintei kanja*) to receive the compensation, the sufferers must prove that they fall into more than two categories below (excluding those who were prenatally exposed to methylmercury in utero): sensory impairment; dyskinesia or motor impairment; equilibration disturbance; concentric contraction of visual field; vision impairment from central nervous system disorder; hearing impairment from central nervous system disorder; and others. The record proves that the category of "patients" was narrowly defined so that Chisso would not go bankrupt by compensating the sufferers. That is to say, the amount of the compensation money paid to an individual was determined not by the degree of damages that people suffer, but by Chisso's capability. See Takamine Takeshi, *Minamatabyō o shitte imasuka* (Tokyo: Iwanami shoten, 2016), 43–47.

Chapter 1

Janaka Shaba or a World Otherwise

MINAMATA AND FUKUSHIMA

The small city of Minamata, located on the southern island of Kyushu in the Japanese archipelago, is known for an industrial disease named after the city. Minamata disease is caused by the ingestion of the methylmercury that was released for more than three decades, beginning in 1937, from a factory owned by the Chisso Corporation. Methylmercury flowed into the Shiranui Sea, where it accumulated in, and eventually damaged or destroyed, the natural environment, including fish and seashells. Human health was also affected by the food chain by this environmental disaster. Once mercury enters the human body and accumulates to a sufficient degree, it affects the nervous system, paralyzing the tongue, fingers, and legs. One eventually loses control of the whole body and often dies an agonizing death.

If death does not come quickly, one is condemned to living with a host of excruciating symptoms for the rest of one's life. Children are especially vulnerable to the effects of mercury. In Minamata, it is estimated that, in the four years between 1955 and 1959, more than 200 prenatally exposed infants were born with the disease.[1] Animals do not escape the effects of this pollution either. Minamata residents have long noticed cats wobbling as they walked, or moving erratically and frenetically, some losing control of themselves, falling into the sea and drowning. Despite widely observed abnormalities surrounding Minamata and the residents' long-held suspicion that the chemicals released by the Chisso Corporation caused fatal diseases, officials did not confirm the causal relation between the disease and Chisso's wastewater for decades.

Thanks to neglect by the corporation, local and national governments, and the medical community, the residents' sufferings became more intense and prolonged. While acknowledging that the life stories of those affected by any environmental destruction differ from one another in the ways in which diseases manifest in their bodies and the manners in which the afflicted bodies are treated, delving into the history of Minamata will reveal similarities to human and ecological suffering in the ongoing aftermath of Fukushima. The intent in comparing Minamata and Fukushima is certainly not to reduce the specificity of either disaster in conflating them, but rather to reveal the common pattern of denial of harm done to human bodies and the environment, as well as the evasion of responsibility by the parties that perpetrated that damage. Focusing on these similarities will allow us to avoid treating Minamata and Fukushima as isolated events, and will instead help us grasp them as the result of shared structural problems.[2] Geographically, both sites are located far from metropolitan areas: Minamata is ninety-five miles from Fukuoka, the largest city on Kyushu Island and close to 600 miles from Tokyo, while the Fukushima Daiichi nuclear power plant is 140 miles from Tokyo. Being in these "peripheral" locations, where the main sources of livelihood are agriculture, forestry, and fishing, rendered the residents financially vulnerable in an era of industrialization. This vulnerability in turn led to the residents' enthusiastically taking employment opportunities at a chemical factory and a nuclear power plant in their respective locations, resulting in a revival of their previously sluggish local economies.

Screenwriter Tani Ken'ichi, who himself grew up in Fukushima, captures the economic despair as well as the hopes placed in the new nuclear industry in this area in the first part of his theatrical trilogy, *1961nen: Yoru ni noboru taiyō* (*1961: Midnight Sunrise*).[3] In this fictive narrative based upon real-life local experiences, TEPCO employers and the Futaba town mayor, Tanaka Seitarō, come to the protagonist's household to cajole his family into selling their land to make way for the construction of a nuclear power plant. Tanaka tries to convince them: "The Northeastern region of Japan is generally poor, but Fukushima is poorer than any other prefecture in the region. Individual incomes are ranked second from the bottom, and the tax income is the worst in the country. Given that, our Futaba area is the poorest in Fukushima."[4] The central government's 1956 Economic White Paper declared "*mohaya sengo dewa nai*" (we are no longer in the postwar period) and indicated that Japan had arisen from the chaotic aftermath of World War I (thanks in part to the Korean War, in which the US military's demands for commodities such as the uniforms and barbed wires helped to renew Japanese fabric and steel industries). Despite these claims that Japan had entered a new phase of economic recovery, areas such as Futaba did not enjoy significant economic advancement.

"Once the nuclear power plant is built," continues Tanaka, "more jobs, and more job security, will be created in our township. We won't have to leave home between farming seasons to take on temporary jobs in the cities. What do you think? Not just that. The plant will bring in the corporate taxes and property taxes, which will allow us to build a library and other facilities so that we can leave some assets to our children and grandchildren. We can turn this unprofitable town into an economically viable one."[5] The nuclear power plant promised a better life to the area's residents for generations to follow, offering a rosy picture to the community. In the end, the town welcomed the nuclear power plant. The promises of TEPCO to the Fukushima community must have resounded ominously for the residents of Minamata, however, who half a century ago welcomed a Chisso factory into their village in order to save it from economic decline. We will return to the history of Minamata in chapter 2, but in the meantime, I shall note some important similarities between the two communities.

The headquarters of both TEPCO and Chisso are located in Tokyo. The products of the respective corporations—TEPCO provides electricity while Chisso makes fertilizer and raw materials for plastic—were distributed and circulated as modern currencies sustaining and advancing Japan's industrialization. Fukushima provided electricity exclusively for the Tokyo metropolitan area, while Minamata's products were widely consumed throughout Japan. The geographical distance between the sites of production and consumption corresponded to and abetted a psychological distance separating residents of Minamata and Fukushima, who suffered on account of the production of plastic and electricity, and those who enjoyed the comforts of those products. Both types of distance in turn allowed for an attitude of indifference to prevail among urbanites intent on maintaining their modern, comfortable mode of living. The geographical and psychological distances between the urban centers and the rural peripheries thus reproduced and reinforced inequitable economic and class relations.

Judith Butler refers to the systemic conditions that produce such inequitable relations as "precarity." According to Butler, while "precariousness" is a shared existential condition (we are all vulnerable in multitudinous ways, needing "food, shelter, and other conditions for persisting and flourishing"),[6] "precarity" is the "politically induced condition that would deny equal exposure [to material and other means for flourishing] through the radically unequal distribution of wealth and the differential ways of exposing certain populations, racially and nationally conceptualized, to greater violence."[7] Butler's analysis suggests that indifference to local sufferings, though *reproduced* by geographical and psychological distances between the urban and the rural, cannot be *reduced* to these distances alone, but are the effect of systemic "precarity." In fact, as we will see, conditions of precarity account for the fact that even within the local population of Minamata, not all people were sympathetic to the victims of Minamata disease.

In Minamata, where the local economy was heavily dependent on the Chisso Corporation—the factory itself as well as the company's subsidiaries—accusations against the corporation were seen by many as a threat to the city's economic life and thus a betrayal. Indeed, around 1967, the citizens' movement to protect Chisso swept through Minamata city, raising the question of whose concerns should prevail: those of the 111 Minamata sufferers or those of the 45,000 Minamata citizens whose economic well-being depended on Chisso.[8] Employees of the corporation discounted or even harassed the sufferers. Even as those employees fell ill one after another, socioeconomic insecurity dissuaded employees from coming forward about their methylmercury poisoning; they feared the very alienation that they had inflicted upon other sufferers. For similar reasons, in Fukushima, voicing concerns about radiation was often discouraged, perceived as threatening to local agriculture and the wider economy, or as a challenge to the safety propaganda promoted by TEPCO, the local and national governments, and some medical professionals.[9]

Towns like Fukushima and Minamata that host major companies are called *kigyō jōkamachi*, literally "corporate castle towns." Residents of a corporate castle town, in cases of disasters caused by the corporation, may find themselves undergoing something like Stockholm syndrome, in which the captive's survival instinct unconsciously develops into an affinity with the captor, even to the point of trying to protect the captor, despite captives being deprived of basic human rights. Perhaps this syndrome is not exclusive to corporate castle towns but characterizes the modern world more broadly. Eventually, the hostage refuses to perceive the situation as imprisonment and instead sees it as a result of her own free will, sometimes expressing gratitude for being allowed to live, even as the captor continues to threaten or damage the hostage's body and environment.

Even as pressure to protect the company comes from within a community, outsiders, too, criticize the victims, suggesting they brought the disaster onto themselves. According to this line of thinking, people in Minamata had invited Chisso to their village and had prospered thanks to its presence there. Thus, these critics assert, there is no ground for complaint. Such rhetoric resurfaced again after Fukusima. Internal and external reproaches for making public the sufferings caused by a corporation made it difficult for the sufferers not only to express their opinions but even to recognize their own precarity. Although their suffering was not accidental but, as Butler reveals, a result of a systemic precarity, some sufferers may have inadvertently internalized the recriminations and denied their own victimhood.

Such imposed silence and self-denial has been characterized by Norma Field, a Japanese studies scholar, as "alienation from one's own victimhood" stemming from the "dissociation of life from livelihood (*seikatsu to seimei no kairi*)."[10] *Seimei* (life) and *seikatsu* (livelihood) should not be separated, yet too often, people find themselves in a situation where they are forced to choose one over the other. The more privileged sectors of a population, thanks to access to both tangible and intangible resources—wealth as well as social connections and the like—can choose life over livelihood. But many others must "choose" livelihood, even when such a choice will harm their lives in the long term. Nevertheless, their choice of livelihood is too often deemed a matter of *jiko sekinin*, or personal responsibility, not the outcome of inequitable social and economic conditions. Inevitably, then, responsibility for the consequences of the "choice" falls to the underprivileged alone—a manifestation of the system of precarity.

Theorists like Butler and Athena Athanasiou attribute the precarity imposed upon the relatively underprivileged majority to today's neoliberal ideology. But the conditions that impel the either/or choice between life and livelihood is not new.[11] The modern understanding of personhood that underlies neoliberalism is itself predicated upon the idea of the individual as an independent and autonomous agent who makes choices based upon free will, and who is, therefore, accountable for the consequences of their choices. This notion of personhood is entrenched in the collective psyche and is fundamental to modern society. Yet, as we can now see, this position contains a contradiction. For those who enjoy more socioeconomic privilege are free *not* to have to choose between life and livelihood, thereby relieving them of responsibility. Then, a disproportionate share of responsibility falls to the relatively underprivileged, who, in "choosing" livelihood over life, are forced to take responsibility for this false choice. As we will see, this unequal distribution of responsibility will be at stake in the lawsuits filed against the executives of Chisso and TEPCO.

In light of the contradiction inherent in the modern conception of personhood, challenging the presupposition that humans are independent and autonomous will be crucial to environmental ethics. Seeking to bring environmental ethics into the political realm, Jane Bennett advocates the notion of the "agency of assemblages," which extends agency to nonhuman, and even nonorganic, beings.[12] That is to say, individual agency is not complete unto itself, uninfluenced by others, but is constituted according to various influences deriving from the existence of other entities, including, for example, "the electrical power grid."[13] Once this extended notion of agency is understood, Bennett argues, our politics must change; it must take up the ethical task of "cultivat[ing] the ability to discern nonhuman vitality, to become perceptually open to it."[14] The Hongan no kai members I treat in this book implicitly understand and employ the concept of the agency of assemblages and its ethical implications; though they express them in different terms and modalities, these individuals envision a world constituted of such extended agencies. They refer to their vision as *janaka shaba*, or what I call "a world otherwise."

HONGAN NO KAI AND JANAKA SHABA

In order to envision the world otherwise—one that challenges the construction of personhood on the basis of individuals' independence and autonomy—examining the lived experiences of the Minamata people, and in particular the members of Hongan no kai, is enlightening.[15] It is from these experiences that *janaka shaba*—a phrase specific to the Minamata dialect—emerges. Minamata resident and sufferer Hamamoto Tsuginori, who later became a founding member of Hongan no kai, introduced this term at the preparatory meeting for the People's Plan 21st Century International People's Action.[16]

In differentiating this notion of a world otherwise from otherworldly concepts like heaven, hell, the kingdom of God, an afterlife, and so on, I borrow an idea from French philosopher Emmanuel Levinas's masterpiece, *Otherwise than Being*. Here Levinas seeks a new mode of existence that breaks free from the Western philosophical tradition of ontology. In his book, Levinas advocates a fundamental shift in the ethical relationship between self and other, one in which the other has primacy over the self.[17] I wish to claim that *janaka shaba* indicates a vision that coincides with the one conceptualized by Levinas in its ethical endeavor to realize relational concept of being in the world that is conceived and constituted in a fundamentally different manner than conventionally and traditionally understood in the modern West. It is in order to preserve the resonance with Levinas's project that I translate the Minamata people's vision as "a world otherwise."

With this in mind, let us examine the inception of the Hongan no kai group. Hongan no kai is one among several groups that have formed in Minamata in response to the disease that has afflicted the city. Hongan no kai was convened by its seventeen founding members, who consisted of Minamata disease sufferers and supporters, including those who I closely examine in this book: the Sugimotos (Eiko and Takeshi), Ogata Masato, and Ishimure Michiko. Focusing on their notions of *nosari* or gift by Sugimoto, *furusato* or home/land by Ishimure, and *shōgoku* or birthplace by Ogata, will illuminate their conception of a world otherwise, brought force by Hongan no kai's *tamashii ishi*, or the stone statues. The group formed in 1994, when media reportage implied that the tragedy of Minamata disease was coming to an end with a court decision to compensate the plaintiffs, a group of sufferers. Despite the fact that several ongoing legal cases had been brought by sufferers, Japanese media suggested that the matter had been overstated, thus motivating the founders of Hongan no kai to organize a group. Contrary to the accounts circulating in the media, Hongan no kai believed that the Minamata issue was far from being resolved. Not only was litigation still under way in other court cases; members of the group felt compelled to address problems that the legal system alone could not adequately resolve.

The term *hongan* means "original vow/s." *Hongan* is commonly associated with the vow made by Amida Buddha to achieve universal salvation. Amida Buddha is worshipped primarily in the Pure Land and True Pure Land schools of Buddhism, the latter of which is prevalent in Minamata and thus familiar to the members of Hongan no kai. Although the group has adopted and adapted Buddhist language, imagery, and rituals, it avoids the dogmatic frameworks of established Buddhism and firmly refuses any institutional religious affiliation. Indeed, Ogata emphasizes that Hongan no kai has no desire to become a religious organization. He explains that the use of the term *hongan* is not intended to tie the group to the "original vow" of Amida Buddhism, but rather derives from the desire "to deepen the idea of *inochi no negai* or 'vow for life.'"[18] Ogata repeatedly makes clear that taking the term *hongan* for the group's name is not to establish institutional allegiance or alliance. On the contrary, the group appropriates and adapts the term *hongan* to reveal the failure of existing organized religions to respond adequately to human suffering of people and to address environmental problems both within and beyond Minamata.

Ogata does not hide his disappointment in the Buddhist temple in Minamata:

> Most villagers identify with the Nishi-Honganji sect [a denomination of True Pure Land Buddhism]. But they are indifferent to the (teaching of) religion except conducting funerals. To them, it is a "funeral Buddhism." The priests, for their part, wouldn't think of lending a hand to help a sick parishioner. Their indifference persisted through and through for the forty years of history of Minamata disease. The villagers were not disturbed (as they had not expected much to begin with). They continued to support the temples but did not place their trust in established religion.[19]

Not only had Buddhist priests and practitioners failed to act; neither Christian ministers nor the Shinto priests in Minamata tried to alleviate the sufferings of the sufferers but, rather, distanced themselves from the sufferers' struggles at the outbreak of the disease.

Hagihara Shūko, a scholar of religion at Kumamoto Gakuin University who examines the ethical responses of Minamata sufferers, explains that Hongan no kai eschews "a consensus on the definitions of such terms as 'soul,' 'life,' or 'prayer,' crucial to their thoughts and actions. Rather, each member continues to ask herself incessantly what these words mean to her."[20] The deliberate choice of avoiding fixed definitions reflects a manifestation of Hongan no kai members' determination to embrace the multidimensional character of our lives. In this regard, Hongan no kai attempts to construe what Edith Wyschogrod terms a "non-nomological ethic."[21] Non-nomological ethics relies not on norms that serve as formulas with universal applications but on the idea that multiple perspectives, values, and dimensions should be recognized (a matter to which we will return). Hongan no kai's ethics emerges from their lived experiences, is firmly rooted in actions, and seeks ways to realize a world otherwise, a world whose modality is fundamentally different from that of this world.

Here, it is important to emphasize that Hongan no kai's envisioned world otherwise must be understood not as an escapist quest for a world that exists only in one's nostalgic fantasies of an idealized premodern society. Rather, their vision points to a new modality of collective life while challenging the modern myth of humans as independent and autonomous; it embraces the fact that we are indebted to other beings for our very lives. In other words, their envisioned world otherwise reveals that the modern view of human beings as independent and autonomous is not only false but indeed harmful, a point underscored by Bennett: "Autonomy and strong responsibility seem to me to be empirically false, and thus their invocation seems tinged with injustice."[22]

Nonetheless, the modern system is founded upon this myth of autonomy, giving rise to a host of problems. Hongan no kai's vision of a world otherwise directs our attention to humans' interdependence, focusing on their shared fragility and vulnerability—our existential "precariousness"—as well as politically induced "precarity." Admitting to and embracing precariousness/precarity enables one to reconceptualize human relationships with other beings and to recognize the inadequacy and inequities of the modern social structure, predicated upon the concept of human autonomy.

MODERNITY, RELIGIOUS SENTIMENT, ETHICALITY

Before proceeding further, it will be helpful to clarify certain key terms integral to this project. The terms "modern" and "modernity" have a wide range of meanings for scholars across various disciplines. For example, sociologist Shoko Yoneyama, the author of *Animism in Contemporary Japan*, notes that sociologists often differentiate the periods before and after 1980; pre-1980 modernity is referred to as "'first' or 'solid' modernity," while post-1980 modernity is defined as the "late/second/liquid modernity."[23] The economic system of post-1980 late-industrial capitalism has been referred to under many different names, often evoking a different salient characteristic. Economist Susan Strange, for example, calls this economic system "casino capitalism";[24] journalist Naomi Klein labels it "disaster capitalism";[25] and philosopher Rob Nixon refers to it as "turbo capitalism."[26]

I have thus far used the term "modern" rather sweepingly, to indicate a complex political, legal, and social system. In situating Minamata's modernization, I draw upon anthropologist Frédérique Apffel-Marglin's discussion of Western modernization. Apffel-Marglin locates the division of the premodern and the modern at the time of the "enclosure movement" in Europe, which constituted the birth of economic privatization.[27] According to Apffel-Marglin, the origin of the modern market economy goes back to the "late fifteenth, sixteenth, seventeenth, and eighteenth centuries" when "the enclosure movement in England particularly, but in other European countries as well," began. Here the "lands previously held in common were forcibly enclosed and 'improved' by a wealthy class that asserted exclusive rights over" such lands.[28]

It was over the course of these centuries that privatization gradually emerged. Along with it came the idea of the human person as an autonomous and independent individual, which in turn formed the basis of modern legal, social, educational, philosophical, religious, ethical, spiritual, and other systems. When such modernization reached Japan in the nineteenth century, it brought with a change in the concept of personhood. Applying Apffel-Marglin's observation of the European context to Japanese modernization, I highlight the following statement: the "transition from the [premodern] gift (or moral) economy to the market economy . . . played a central role in the de-spiriting of the non-human world"[29] and thereby changed human relations not only with other humans but with nonhumans and other-than-humans, as well. "Other-than-humans" is Apffel-Marglin's term for entities that "[embody] both human and non-human aspects."[30] Other-than-humans include such things as deities, gods, ogres, demons, and *tamashii*, or spirit, a concept that is quite familiar to people in Minamata.

In the context of the Japanese archipelago, according to medievalist Sakurai Eiji, at least for the time period from the late fifteenth century to the early sixteenth century, the gift economy and the market economy coincided and were quite close to each other in their practices.[31] But a more rapid and drastic shift took place in the nineteenth century as a result of encountering the Western system of modernity. At the inception of the modern nation-state of Japan, various transformations—social, political, and economic—were rewriting people's relations: relationships with fellow humans, nonhumans, and other-than-humans.

The transition to the market economy, as Apffel-Marglin claims, changed humans' perception of themselves, of others (nonhumans and other-than-humans), and of their surroundings, which in turn affected humans' interactions with each other. Such changes instigated a shift in ethics, as well. In a conversation with Claude Levi-Strauss, philosopher Nakazawa Shin'ichi, referring to Native Americans' religious cultures, argued that the notion of the gift serves as the ground for ethical relations between humans and nature.[32] The absolute power of nature—for better and worse—evokes feelings of gratitude and fear in humans. Gratitude is expressed in ritual offerings expressing hope for nature's continuous blessings, while fear finds expression in rituals of pacification or forgiveness. To the modern sensibility, which fails to appreciate the agency of other-than-humans, such rituals may appear "irrational," but they serve as a reminder of humans' precarious condition in the world.

Academia has, too, been a force in the modern disenchant of the world.[33] Feminist theorist AnaLouise Keating comments on the eschewal of other-than-humans that prevails in much academic discourse in terms that bear on our study here. She describes the concept of "spiritual activism" advocated and practiced by author and activist Gloria E. Anzaldúa: "Beliefs and practices consciously making reference to the s/Spirit as the common life force within and between all beings are largely marginalized from serious intellectual discourse as superstition, folk belief, or New Age delusion when they are not relegated to the socially controlled spaces of the orientalist study of 'primitive animism' or of 'respectable' religion within dominant culture."[34]

In pointing out such matters, I do not mean to suggest that restoring our belief in other-than-human beings would be a solution to the problems of modernity. Nor do I advocate a nostalgic return to a premodern mentality, or a restoration of lost religious faith or spirituality. Rather, I seek to articulate and condone the environmental ethics evident in the thought and practice of Hongan no kai, which suggests that retrieving or reconstruing the agency of humans, nonhumans, and other-than-humans, may provide a practical mode of resistance to the degradations wrought by the modern economic system. It is this alternative worldview of Hongan no kai is what they call *janaka shaba*—a world otherwise. Realizing this world otherwise, Hongan no kai insists, is an urgent ethical task.

In articulating and enabling the pursuit of this ethical task, I frequently draw upon Wyschogrod's definition of ethics: "Ethics is the sphere of transactions between 'self' and 'Other.'"[35] Echoing Levinas, Wyschogrod's definition does not center on the self but on relationality, acknowledging the others' import in the formation of the self. Building on Wyschogrod, and in resistance to much traditional philosophical discourse in the West, I conceive of the category of the "other" to include not only other human beings but also nonhumans and other-than-humans. Wyschogrod continues: "(Ethics) is to be construed non-nomologically, it cannot look to traditional philosophical discourse for a perspective on human conduct."[36] Ethics does not connote a formula assuming universal applicability; rather, ethics refers to the opening of oneself to many possibilities and potentials in the world, going beyond one's habitual horizon. Adapting Wyschogrod's concept of ethics in this manner, it becomes clear that Hongan no kai's praxis—their thoughts and actions—constitutes an ethical task, as they demonstrate ways to envision and to realize possibilities and potentials for reconceiving one's relations with all other beings in a world otherwise.

Envisioning such a world—open, multivalent, and multidimensional—constitutes a critical response to problems rooted in "precarity." Living in a world dominated by market values, we are also culturally conditioned to blind ourselves to precarity, tending to ignore humans and others who do not uphold or participate in the de-spirited world of the marketplace. Judith Butler's writings on post 9-11 America offer insight into what prevents recognition of precarity. She asks, "What are the cultural barriers against which we struggle when we attempt to name, and so to bring under the rubric of the 'human,' those whom the United States and its allies have killed?"[37] Similarly, we may ask what barriers prevented recognition of Minamata sufferers. The modern economic market, which devalues certain humans, has also diminished recognition of a spirited world. The modern system, as Hongon no kai makes clear, does not have the resources for resolving the sufferings and injustice that have emerged as a result of the very conditions it has created. It is in the hope of responding to these sufferings that Hongon no kai seeks to cultivate recognition of a world otherwise.

THE RELIGIOUS SENSIBILITY OF HONGAN NO KAI

Hongan no kai's efforts arose from the question of how we might envision and realize a world otherwise that operates in a manner that counters the anthropocentrism of the modern world. Their imaginings of such a world, as the name of the group suggests, often draw upon religious language and motifs, but as we have noted, members adamantly refuse to be associated with any religious organizations. They eschew formal, institutional affiliations precisely because their vision remains outside the purview of this world. At the same time, the language and tropes they embrace are those that the modern world has marginalized, excluded, or dismissed as "otherworldly."

One example of this simultaneous refusal of institutional religion and embrace of religious language comes from Ogata Masato, a Minamata fisher, a sufferer, and a founding member of Hongan no kai. Asked to identify the origin of the tragedy in Minamata, he replied: "It may have come from Buddha's back." This enigmatic answer surprised Ogata himself. Referring to a religious figure does not indicate that Ogata, who offers no commentary on this curious reference to Buddha, understands Minamata disease in an "official" Buddhist context. Rather, Ogata uses "Buddha" as a symbol of something other-than-human, a force capable of disrupting the prevailing values and norms of this world. Ogata's response exemplifies his ethics, in which the "good" represented by Buddha and the "bad" associated with the methylmercury poisoning and the irresponsibility of the Chisso Corporation share a common origin.

Further elaborating upon his response, Ogata wonders whether good and evil are not opposing ends of a linear spectrum, but rather moving points along a closed loop. "The closer the relations are, the more intense hatred becomes. Hate and love do not fundamentally differ but might have the same root. When one walks straight from the South Pole, one will eventually reach the North Pole. Thus, everything is connected." "It is true," continues Ogata, "that my home, the Shiranui Sea, was chosen as a place where evil landed. However, precisely because evil lands on this place, it has to be the place where a deity descends. We will have to bring a deity into being."[38] Ogata's apparent conflation of good and evil does not mark a collapse of the foundation of morality. Rather, in imagining the manifestation of a deity—an embodiment of a value system at variance with that of the modern world—Ogata opens the way to a spirited world otherwise.

For Ogata, to exit the market-driven world of modernity and to enter this multivalent, many-spirited world otherwise does not entail abandoning or escaping this world. The world he envisions is neither independent nor autonomous—not a world apart—but, rather, a world open, emerging through the coexistence of multiple values: "To think of good and evil as either/or makes it difficult to imagine living in two worlds simultaneously."[39] Ogata finds a "spiritual community" inhering in this present world. "The spiritual community," he explains, "is like an old-fashioned country stew, in which each person has a different face, physique, character, and age. Some would be disabled and others not. Regardless of their characteristics, all would have valuable roles to play. No one would be expendable. In such a society, there would be no discrimination. To acknowledge each other's differences is to acknowledge our essential equality."[40]

The noninstitutional religious sensibility of Hongan no kai members is further evidenced by their use of the term *tamashii*, or spirit, as found in the title of their newsletter, *Tamashii utsure* (*Transferring the spirit*). According to Ishimure Michiko, the modern world's exclusion of tamashii accounts for its flaws. She writes, "Everyone talks about environmental issues these days, yet no one acknowledges tamashii. What shall we do about this oversight?"[41] In order to avoid further environmental disaster, Ishimure insists that we should shift our anthropocentric view to a more inclusive one that embraces nonhumans and other-than-humans, including spirits.

Ogata, too, discusses tamashii, explaining that tamashii are a functional life force. "From a modern perspective, there is no such a thing as an afterlife but only [a] void after one's death." Yet, Ogata does not believe that one's existence ends with the death of the body: "Life has two dimensions. One is a life that is corporeal, gone with one's physical body [upon death]. The other is a life that is functional. Even after one's body perishes and decays, its function will stay. That is why we hold anniversary rituals for the dead. The function of life is eternal."[42] Tamashii are this eternal source of life—this life force. By such an understanding, tamashii are afforded agency that affects the living. To modern ears, the religious rhetoric of Hongan no kai's members may sound irrational or incomprehensible—a nebulous mysticism. But framing the activity of tamashii in functional terms suggests a view of the world—this present, earthly world—in which the dead are not relegated to an otherworldly plane, a matter borne out by the fact that commemoration of the dead is an integral part of sustaining the modern nation-state, as noted by many scholars.[43] In this respect, modern society is not as "secular" as it aspires to be (a matter to which we will return below).

Thus far, I have introduced some key concepts for understanding Hongan no kai's praxis. Although I am fascinated by Hongan no kai, I do not personally share all their beliefs. I suspect the same will be the case with most readers of this book. I do, however, wish to recognize the value of their concrete efforts to redress the problems of the modern world. For the moment, I recommend pausing before judging their thoughts and actions as misguided or insufficient to the ethical task they seek to address. Indeed, I take this willing suspension of judgment to be a crucial moment in genuine ethical thinking. We should allow our usual modes of judgment to be interrupted for a moment as we move forward in contemplating the group's enigmatic statements seemingly incomprehensible actions and thereby begin the self-critical task of evaluating and reevaluating our own ethical thoughts and conduct. Learning about Hongan no kai's praxis in the following pages may provide readers the occasion to imagine a world in which multifaceted and unfamiliar values coexist.

NOTES

1. Harada Masazumi and Tajiri Masami, "Shounisei · taijisei Minamatabyō ni kansuru rinshou ekigakuteki kenkyū" (An epidemiological and clinical study of infantile and congenital Minamata disease: A consideration of the effect of methyl mercury on fetal and infantile development), *Department of Social Welfare Studies* 14, no. 1 (2009): 6.

2. The methylmercury poisoning again took place in Niigata in 1965, and the Fukushima accident was certainly not the first nuclear disaster in Japan.

3. *1961nen: Yoru ni noboru taiyō* (1961: Midnight sunrise), written and directed by Tani Ken'ichi, Iwaki Performing Arts Center Alios, July 8, 2018. I was able to see this performance of the play.

4. Tani, *1961nen*, scenario 34.
5. Tani, *1961nen*, scenario 34.
6. Judith Butler, *Frames of War: When Is Life Grievable?* (London: Verso, 2009), 28–29.
7. Butler, *Frames of War*, 28.
8. Koga, Tōru, *Risei no bōryoku: Nihonshakai no byōrigaku* (Violence by reason: Pathology of Japanese society) (Tokyo: Seitousha, 2014), 245.
9. Oyabu, Junko, "Fukushima genpatsujiko kara 8nenme 'hinansha o shiensuru hinansha' wa nani o omou" (8 years have passed since Fukushima nuclear accident: What is in mind of "the evacuees who support other evacuees"?), *Diamond online*, August 24, 2018 (https://diamond.jp/articles/-/178130?page=4). This example is an online report about the evacuees' difficulties voicing their concerns about radiation exposure.
10. Norma, Field, "'Heiwa to han'ei' no ato de: Shikago daigaku meiyo kyoju Norma Field-san ni kiku" (After "Peace and Prosperity": Interview with Norma Field, Professor Emerita, University of Chicago), *Asahi Shimbun,* March 1, 2014.
11. Judith Butler and Athena Athanasiou, *Dispossession: The Performative in the Political* (Malden, MA: Polity, 2013), 103–108.
12. Jane Bennett, *Vibrant Matter: A Political Ecology of Things* (Durham, NC: Duke University Press, 2010), 37. While Bennett acknowledges that nonhumans affect humans' lives as vital materiality, I am uncertain as to whether she would be comfortable with the notion of the other-than-human agent.
13. Bennett, *Vibrant Matter*, 20–24.
14. Bennett, *Vibrant Matter*, 14.
15. Their newsletter, *Tamashii utsure* (*Transferring the spirit*) introduces the English name as "Club of the Original Vow," but I took the liberty here of translating it as "Association," reflecting the group's relaxed friendship among the members and their activities.
16. Hanazaki, Kōhei, *"Janaka shaba" no tetsugaku: jendā, esunishitī, ekologī* (Philosophy of "*Janaka shaba*": Gender, ethnicity, and ecology) (Tokyo: Inpakuto shuppankai, 2002), 96. Hanazaki, Kōhei explains the term and vision of *janaka shaba* as follows: "At the preparatory meeting for the People's Plan 21st Century International People's Action, members discussed an alternative society, so people would be able to choose their lifestyles according to their life patterns and beliefs. Then, Hamamoto Tsuginori, who was working with Minamata disease sufferers, uttered that such an alternative society is, in our dialect, *janaka shaba*—the world operated otherwise."
17. Emmanuel Levinas, *Otherwise than Being of Beyond Essence*, trans. Alphonso Lingis (Norwell, MA: Kluwer Academic Publishers, 1991), 11–12.
18. Ogata, Masato, "Hongan no kai zadankai Inochi no negai o oimotomete" (Hongan no kai roundtable: seeking for the vow of life) *Tamashii utsure*, 36 (2009): 7.
19. Ogata, Masato, *Rowing the Eternal Sea: The Story of a Minamata Fisherman,* interview by Oiwa Keibo, trans. by Karen Collingan-Taylor (Lanham, MD: Rowman & Littlefield Publishers, 2001), 171.

20. Hagihara, Shūko, "Umiotosareru kotoba, tewatasareteiku kotoba: Minamatabyō jiken to 'Hongan no kai'" (Words brought forth, words handed down: the Minamata disease incident and "Hongan no kai"), *Shūkyō kenkyū,* 86, no. 2 (2012): 209 (399).

21. Edith Wyschogrod, *Saints and Postmodernism: Revisioning Moral Philosophy* (Chicago: The University of Chicago Press, 1990), xv. "Ethics is the sphere of transactions between 'self' and 'Other' and is to be construed non-nomonologically."

22. Bennett, *Vibrant Matter*, 37.

23. Shoko Yoneyama, *Animism in Contemporary Japan: Voices for the Anthropocene from Post-Fukushima Japan* (New York: Routledge, 2019). In terms of the definition of modernity, see Shoko Yoneyama, "Life-world: Beyond Fukushima and Minamata," *Japan Focus: Asia-Pacific Journal* 10, no. 42 (2) (2012). https://apjjf.org/2012/10/42/Shoko-YONEYAMA/3845/article.html The terms "late modern," "second modern," and "liquid modern" are coined by Anthony Giddens, *Modernity and Self-Identity: Self and Society in the Late Modern Age* (Stanford: Stanford University Press, 1991); Ulrich Beck, *World Risk Society* (Cambridge: Polity, 1999); and Zygmunt Bauman, *Liquid Modernity* (Cambridge: Polity, 2000), respectively.

24. Susan Strange, *Casino Capitalism* (Manchester: Manchester University Press, 1997), especially 1–3.

25. Naomi Klein, *The Shock Doctrine: The Rise of Disaster Capitalism* (New York: Picador, 2007).

26. Rob Nixon, *Slow Violence and the Environmentalism of the Poor* (Cambridge, MA: Harvard University Press, 2011), 8.

27. Apffel-Marglin, *Subversive Spiritualities*, 36.

28. Apffel-Marglin, *Subversive Spiritualities*, 36.

29. Apffel-Marglin, *Subversive Spiritualities*, 16.

30. Apffel-Marglin, *Subversive Spiritualities*, 11. Timothy Morton also suggests an interrelationship among fife forms and those of nonlife: "This is a momentous era, at which we achieve what has sometimes been called *ecological awareness.* Ecological awareness is a detailed and increasing sense, in science and outside of it, of the innumerable interrelationships among lifeforms and between life and non-life." Timothy Morton, *Hyperobjects: Philosophy and Ecology after the End of the World* (Minneapolis, MI: University of Minnesota Press, 2013), 128.

31. Sakurai, Eiji, *Zouyo no rekishigaku: Girei to keizai no aida* (Historiography of the gift: Between courtesy and economy) (Tokyo: Chūō kōron shinsha, 2011), iii and 172–173.

32. Nakazawa, Shin'ichi, *Wakusei no fūkei: Nakazawa Shin'ichi taidanshū* (The Scenery of the planet: Conversations with Nakazawa Shin'ichi) (Tokyo: Seidosha, 2014), 49.

33. Max Weber, "Science as a Vocation," *Daedalus*, 87, no. 1 (1958): 133.

34. AnaLouise Ketain, "'I'm a Citizen of the Universe': Gloria Anzalúa's Spiritual Activism as Catalyst for Social Change," *Feminist Studies* 34, no. 1/2 (2008): 54.

35. Wyschogrod, *Saints and Postmodernism*, xv.

36. Wyschogrod, *Saints and Postmodernism*, xv.

37. Judith Butler, *Precarious Life: The Powers of Mourning and Violence* (London: Verso, 2004), 46.

38. Ogata, Masato and Tsuji, Shinichi, *Tokoyo no fune o kogite* (Rowing the eternal sea) (Yokohama: Seori shobō, 1996), 218–219.

39. Ogata, Masato, "Hontou no 'kuni' o motomete" (Seeking for a true home), *Gonzui*, no. 95 (2006): 94.

40. Ogata and Tsuji, *Tokoyo no fune o kogite*, 172.

41. Ishimure, Michiko, *Soseishita tamashii o nosete* (On board with the resurrected spirit) (Tokyo: Kawaide shobō shinsha, 2013), 108.

42. Ogata, "Hontou no 'kuni' o motomete," 94.

43. For example, Harry Harootunian, "Memory, Mourning, and National Morality: Yasukuni Shrine and the Reunion of State and Religion in Postwar Japan," in *Nation and Religion: Perspectives on Europe and Asia*, eds. by Peter Van Der Veer and Hartmut Lehmann (Princeton, NJ: Princeton University Press, 1999), 144–160.

Chapter 2

Modernization, Mercury, and Minamata

Timothy S. George opens his monumental book *Minamata* by taking the reader on a journey from metropolitan Tokyo to the once booming but now rather quiet city of Minamata, on Kyūshū Island.[1] From a train window, the route offers alternately bucolic and industrial scenes. In the time since George penned his description, Minamata has constructed a bullet train station, Shin-Minamata (2004). From this stop, it is another ten-minute taxi ride, or one stop on the Hisatsu Orenji line of the local train, to reach the old Minamata station. Across the street from this station, the well-maintained and modern buildings of the Japan New Chisso (JNC) factory, in stark contrast to the modest appearance of Minamata station, stretch out, occluding the view of the Shiranui Sea. The JNC is now known for its production of the liquid crystals that are integral components for the displays of TVs, computers, and cell phones—so many "essentials" of modern life. The JNC itself is new, established in 2011 as separate from its holding company, the Chisso Corporation.

In this chapter, I will unpack the history of Chisso from its inception through 1960 and its relation to Minamata's development, examining its influence on the people of Minamata. On our way to examining the vision of a world otherwise enacted by Hongan no kai members, I describe the general attitude of Minamata residents toward the sufferers, who in turn will facilitate our understanding of the background of this alternative vision of the world. The goal of my account is not to demonize Chisso or those who did not support the sufferers. Rather, it is to demonstrate the complex social strata and living conditions of Minamata, thanks to which many citizens who were affected by the ingestion of methylmercury were unable to recognize the violence done to their own bodies, their livelihoods, the community, and the environment. This chapter thus serves as a bridge between chapter 1, which laid out the ethical framework of this book, and the following chapters, which will investigate individual cases as responses to the sufferers' maltreatment by their fellow citizens, the local and central governments, and Chisso.

To this end, I consider modernization in Minamata by examining the biography of Chisso's founder, Noguchi Shitagau, then trace Chisso's expansion as a part of the colonial project of the Japanese Empire, demonstrating that economic growth at this time was made possible by the exploitation of laborers and colonized land. This concise historical survey will serve as a context for considering the plight of Minamata sufferers and the prolongation of their struggles. However, this is not a cut-and-dried case of Chisso versus the people; the matter is complex, for employees of the corporation implicated during this time were not a monolithic entity. Initially, Chisso's employees tended to view the Minamata sufferers as accusers of the company. Employees, in particular, Chisso's Minamata factory workers, understood themselves as victims, not victimizers. But over time, some of those workers would come to collaborate with the Minamata sufferers. This discussion will allow us, in chapters to follow, to dwell on a more detailed description of Minamata disease, and to consider the sufferers' plights and struggles against discrimination, as well as the stories and legal actions taken by individuals who later became founding members of Hongan no kai.

In the historiographical description to follow, rather than emphasizing transformations of Japan following its defeat, in 1945, of World War II, I focus on the epistemological framework that occluded the precariousness of lives both within and beyond Minamata, and thus contributed to persistent precarity. The overview of Japan's modernization in this regard enables us to see Minamata disease and the turmoil it produced not as an exceptional accident but rather as the inevitable consequence of a failing modern system that creates and maintains an attitude that treats humans, nonhumans, and other-than-humans merely as resources to be exploited—the condition of precarity. In carrying out my analysis, I focus on two particular sets of relationships: first, between Chisso and the city of Minamata; and second, between Chisso's employees and fishers. Examining these relationships across this chapter will allow us to discern the external forces bearing on Minamata as well as the internal struggles out of which the sufferers' ethical praxis emerged.

MINAMATA'S MODERNIZATION AND NOGUCHI SHITAGAU

"Minamata represents and encompasses all the problems posed by Japan's modernization,"[2] Ishimure Michiko observes. Livia Monnet, a scholar known for her nuanced translation of Ishimure's *Kugai jōdo: Waga Minamatabyō*, or *Paradise in the Sea of Sorrow: Our Minamata Disease*, explains Ishimure's indictment of modernity: Ishimure's writings serve "as a critique of modernity and its colonizing, destructive machines and institutions—modern time and modern industrial capitalism, the modern nation-state, and finally the modern discourses of science and technology."[3] Although modernity is a condition, as acclaimed historian of Japan, Carol Gluck has shown,[4] modernization is always a process of *becoming* "modern," which in Japan has entailed catching up with and adopting the North American and Western European modality of modernization. In this way, modernization is synonymous with Westernization. In this chapter, I focus on "modernity" as it has affected Minamata in particular, beginning with the establishment of Chisso.

Hongan no kai member Ogata Masato, whose life will be examined in chapter 4, links Japan's modernization and the problems it wrought to the establishment of Chisso:

> Chisso represents modernization, but we are all modernized, too. . . . Take a look at the case of Minamata disease: The Minamata sufferers have to obtain the government's certification to be recognized as patients, otherwise no medical aid is provided; [in order to compel Chisso to acknowledge their wrongdoings] the sufferers have to file a lawsuit against Chisso and the government—all procedures tied to modernity. Meanwhile, humans are misperceived as mere things, trapped in the system. We are "domesticated" in this system.[5]

By Ogata's account, the arrival of Chisso marks the advent of modernization, with its attendant problems, in Minamata.

The fact that Chisso began as an electric power company is also illuminating. Anthropologist Dominic Boyer writes, "Electricity is a fascinating subject of inquiry because it is in many respects the foundational apparatus upon which the experience of modernity has been constituted since the late nineteenth century."[6] Electricity and modernization are indeed closely linked in Japan. Electricity allowed industries to operate at a large scale, which in turn transformed the makeup of the Japanese labor force, which now included a growing population of factory workers. For reasons that will become clear, it is noteworthy that Chisso's founder, Noguchi Shitagau, began his entrepreneurial career with the construction of a hydropower plant for generating electricity.

Sociologist Yoshimi Shun'ya calls attention to the sudden increase of electricians in the United States in the nineteenth century,[7] a pattern also observable in the modernization of Japan, where the "foundational apparatus" of electricity coincided with a quest for energy motivated by Japan's nation-building and imperialist aspirations. For example, Emperor Meiji, newly enthroned in 1868, at the outset of Japan's modernization, would make six tours through the Japanese archipelago between 1872 and 1885. His tours had dual purposes, both enabled by electricity: first, to create a spectacle by which to impress his sovereign power upon his subjects' minds; and, second, to suppress the anti-Meiji government movement.[8] The scale and success of these tours were owed in part to the use of electricity. Once the emperor's itinerary was established, the government created a telegraph network linking destinations on the tours; telegraph posts, set up for emergencies, granted the emperor a security system that would not have been possible without this electronic medium of communication. This security allowed the emperor to display himself in an unprecedented manner. No longer hidden within a palace in Kyoto, Emperor Meiji traveled among the people, appearing in Western-style military garb. Thanks to electricity, the emperor's tour, with all its pageantry, acted to spectacularly display the emperor's sovereign power and thereby intimidate his anti-Meiji opponents. In turn, the emperor's expeditions facilitated the implementation of electrical transmission lines in Japan.

As was often the case in other countries, the initial reaction toward electricity in Japan was ambivalent; efforts to make sense of electricity found people attributing this strange new power to a supernatural force, whether divine or demonic.[9] But thanks to its widespread dissemination and thus normalization, electricity quickly became a symbol of modern Western civilization. By the Taisho Era (1912–1926), *bunka* (culture/civilization) and *bunka seikatsu* (civilized lifestyle)—a lifestyle represented by the household use of electricity—had become popular phrases.[10] To consume the excess power generated by the proliferation of electric companies, these companies promoted the use of electricity in private homes, propelling the production of electric home appliances.[11] Over time, competition among electric companies became intense,[12] leading to friction, even riots.[13] Even in the years of the economic depression in Japan that followed upon the Great Depression, the demand for electric power continued to increase by twenty percent every year.[14]

Given electricity's role in people's lives and its contribution to economic growth and the expansion of the Japanese empire in the late nineteenth and the first half of the twentieth century, the founder of Chisso, Noguchi Shitagau, then a young and ambitious graduate of Tokyo Imperial University, had the foresight to launch his career in the energy industry in Fukushima. Noguchi was born in Kanazawa, north of Kyoto, in 1873, to a samurai family.[15] Noguchi's father, Yukinobu, who had served the Kaga clan in present-day Kanazawa during the feudal era of the Tokugawa period, moved to Tokyo after the *han* (domain) system was abolished by the newly established Meiji government. In Tokyo, Yukinobu found new employment with the Ministry of Education, a job that enabled his children to receive the best education available at the time.

Thanks to his father's position with the Ministry that enabled him to receive good education, Shitagau was admitted to Japan's only school of engineering during this time, the Faculty of Engineering at Tokyo Imperial

University.[16] While still a student, Noguchi had a part-time job at the electricity plant in Numagami, which supplied the Kōriyama Silk Reeling Company with electricity.[17] It was also during this time that Noguchi witnessed firsthand the growing demand for electricity and the urgent need for a long-distance transmission system to make electricity available in distant locales.

After his graduation, Noguchi continued to work in the electricity industry, now as a chief engineer for the Kōriyama Electric Light Company in Fukushima.[18] His future career seemed as promising as that of any other alumnus of Tokyo Imperial University at the time, but his prospects changed with his father's unexpected death in 1898. As the eldest son of the family, Noguchi was responsible for supporting his mother and younger siblings, which obliged him to return to Tokyo. Although he was able to secure a job at an American trading company immediately upon his return, he soon quit the job, which he found unexciting, and opened an ink retail shop. But the shop did not survive for long. Following the shop's closure, Noguchi settled at the Japanese branch of the German Siemens Company, which was Europe's largest manufacturer at the time producing electrical equipment.[19] The business connections Noguchi established while working for Siemens would come to play a crucial role in expanding his company. Siemens's advanced electrical machinery impressed Noguchi, who stayed with the company until 1901.[20] This job indeed set the course for Noguchi's future entrepreneurial endeavors. For while working for Siemens Noguchi continued to study ways to make use of the calcium carbide generated from the production electricity—an idea that had been percolating since his time in Kōriyama.[21]

Calcium carbide is an electrochemical compound that was in high demand at this time, for when combined with water, it produces acetylene gas, which was used in the lamps that were swiftly spreading throughout Japan. Calcium carbide, along with other synthetics being produced during this period, is also used in nitrogenous fertilizers—the first product that Chisso would eventually manufacture.[22] Noguchi was fascinated by the possibilities of the multiple uses of calcium carbide. When he resigned from Siemens in 1901, he worked briefly as a consultant for the railroad business and the mining industry. Still, his curiosity about chemistry remained undiminished, leading him to make a trip around Europe and America to learn more about science and technology during the outbreak of the Russo-Japanese War of 1904.

After returning from his trip abroad, Noguchi was ready to start a new business. He founded his own electricity company, with help from the friends he had made and connections he had cultivated while working at Siemens and other companies.[23] Among those friends were Nagasato Yūhachi and Hino Tatsuji, who were managing a gold mine in Kagoshima, on southern Kyūshū Island. They convinced Noguchi of the need for additional electric generators for the mines. The conversations with Nagasato and Hino inspired Noguchi to look for a location for the construction of a hydraulic power station in Kyūshū. Noguchi eventually found a waterfall suitable for generating hydroelectricity in the Sogi area of Kagoshima, and thus ideal for a power plant to supply electricity for the gold mine.

Utilizing the knowledge and experience he had acquired at Siemens, Noguchi was able to open Sogi Electric Inc. for operation on January 12, 1906.[24] To his delight, Sogi Electric generated more electricity than expected, with the surplus allowing him to produce more electrochemical products on the side. The more electricity the plant generated, the more subproducts were made for sale, in turn incentivizing Noguchi to produce more electrical power. Eventually, Noguchi began to lay plans for another factory for electrochemical products. In 1907, with his friends Fujiyama Tsuneichi and Ichikawa Seiji, and with capital to the tune of 200,000 yen, Noguchi established a second company, a little north of Sogi, in a small village called Minamata: Nihon Kābaido Shōkai (Japan Carbide Company).[25]

Timothy S. George notes that Minamata residents enthusiastically courted Noguchi's new business for Minamata: "Maeda Eiki, a member of a Minamata samurai family, formed a group of leading citizens to draw Noguchi's interests so as to lure his factory into Minamata."[26] There were three key reasons for Minamata's residents to show such enthusiasm for bringing Noguchi's business to their village. First, Minamata was experiencing a serious economic downturn following upon the Meiji government's change to its taxation system; payments were no longer to be made in rice and other materials, but rather in monetary currency. The rural economy of Minamata had not yet adjusted to this new currency-based taxation system. The wide circulation of electricity was the second reason for their economic hardship. Electricity gradually reduced the demand for candle wax—one of Minamata's main manufactured goods. Finally, the most serious blow to Minamata's economy came with the Russo-Japanese war: sea salt was the other main product coming out of Minamata, but the government monopolized salt in 1905 to cover the immense expense of the war, thereby depriving Minamata of a key source of income.

In addition to these factors, Minamata's importance as a shipping port was on the decline. As the coal mines on Kyūshū Island grew, Minamata Bay proved insufficient to accommodate the scale of the coal trade.[27] When Minamata's main products—wax and salt—dwindled, and with its port becoming irrelevant with the emergence of large-scale industry, the villagers became desperate to host a new industry to help ensure economic survival.

With the help of substantial investments from his business connections, Noguchi managed to keep the companies afloat. Following a few critical months of hardship, Noguchi's Minamata company, Nihon Kābaido Shōkai, began to make profits from carbide production and acetylene from the excess of Sogi Electric, and "became Japan's largest production operations for calcium carbide, using in 1907 a 500-kilowatt electric furnace, yielding 15 tons per month."[28] In addition to substantial financial investments, the success of Nihon Kābaido Shōkai was also attributed to the relationships Noguchi cultivated while working for Siemens, which led to his obtaining a patent for exclusive use of the German technology for production of calcium cyanamide for fertilizer in Japan.[29]

In 1908, Noguchi combined his two companies, Sogi Electric in Sogi, Kagoshima, and Nihon Kābaido Shōkai, in Minamata, Kumamoto. They became Nihon Chisso Hiryō, or Japan Nitrogenous Fertilizers (hereafter Nitchitsu, which will be the company's name until 1945, which becomes Chisso). The newly amalgamated company now produced calcium cyanamide for fertilizer in addition to electricity. Demand for food in response to the population increase across Japan was soaring, and fertilizers were indispensable for augmenting the agricultural yield. Initially, however, Nitchitsu fertilizer sales were not strong, and the company fell into debt. Several factors account for the early sluggishness: the product had a strong, odd smell; farmers knew that calcium cyanamide could be harmful if not used properly; and farmers hesitated to use synthetic chemicals. The hardship continued when Noguchi turned to ammonium sulfate as a substitute for calcium cyanamide, as it met with the same resistance.

Fujiyama, Noguchi's longtime business partner, innovated an inexpensive method for the production of fertilizer in 1911 and saved the company from its growing debt. But the following year, Noguchi and Fujiyama parted ways. Historian Barbara Molony describes Noguchi as "the leader, coming up with new products ahead of its competitor and manufacturing old products by cheaper, more efficient methods,"[30] while Fujiyama, a scientist who found his pleasure in study and research, lacked business acumen. In running the company, Noguchi, ever the entrepreneur, continued to invest aggressively in the company. To the benefit of his company, Noguchi's ambitions were to find support in those of the expanding the Empire of Japan.

The outbreak of World War I in Europe and its aftermath benefited Noguchi's company. As trade in European products were halted with the war, Nitchitsu became the sole provider for domestic demand for fertilizer. Noguchi invented a new nitrogen-fixation method that led to increased profits, giving him yet another business opportunity poised for expansion. In tandem with Noguchi's growing business, Minamata expanded, too, growing from a village of nineteen communities in 1889 to a town with a population of 20,000 in 1912.[31] In the decades to follow, the population continued to rise: "30,000 in 1941, 40,000 in 1948, and a peak of 50,000 in 1956."[32]

George reports that the "Nitchitsu group included 48 companies by April 1941," making Minamata a typical "company castle town." By this time,

Nitchitsu was recognized as a "*kontserun*, (from the German word, Konzern) and one of the 'new conglomerates' (*shinkō zaibatsu*)."[33] The rapid rise of Noguchi's conglomerate has been addressed by writers and scholars. Noguchi's biographer Kamoi Yū, for example, emphasizes that it was not merely fortuitous events and connections, but Noguchi's talent, dedication, and hard work that accounted for the success of his companies.[34] Historian Aaron Stephen Moore, though not discounting Noguchi's work ethic, attributes the success of Nitchitsu to its important role in the Japanese empire's agenda to promote economic growth and military expansion at the time.[35]

Sociologist Fukai Jun'ichi's work supplements Moore's analysis. Fukai points out that the emergence and rapid growth of the new zaibatsu, including Nitchitsu, in the 1920s and 1930s derived from the demands and support of the military industry. The new zaibatsu manufactured materials for combat—explosives, special paint for aircraft fuselages, coal liquefaction, refined aluminum, man-made fiber, and so on—a niche market that the old zaibatsu had not yet exploited.[36] Working with the military government, Nitchitsu, like other new conglomerates, was able to expand. The impact of collaboration with the military was felt in Minamata. Taue Yoshiharu, a Minamata sufferer and a founding member of Hongan no kai, attests that, in his youth, he was mobilized to work for a Nitchitsu plant that was producing military equipment.[37] Thus, in the minds of the residents of Minamata, the increased cash flow, the circulation of electricity, and industrial expansion were all thanks to Nitchitsu and the military government that was driving modernization.

THE COLONIAL EXPERIENCE AND MINAMATA

As we have seen, modernization in Japan was inseparable from the shift to a currency economy, industrial growth, and military expansion. These changes set the stage for the Japanese empire's encroachment on neighboring countries (in the Sino-Japan War in 1894 and the Russo-Japan War in 1904 and beyond). Nitchitsu expanded along with the empire's military and colonization projects. Kamoi's biography of Noguchi, published during his lifetime, glorifies the entrepreneur's expansion of business into the Korean Peninsula as a "discovery of Korea" (*Chōsen hakken*), holding up his achievements as greater than the accomplishments of the governor-general in Korea.[38] It is clear, however, that Noguchi's "discovery" of, and expansion into, Korea is not attributable to his ambition and business skills alone but was largely enabled by the Japanese government.

Prior to the 1930s, few Japanese investors had any interest in Korea, even though Japan had been exploiting people in the Korean Peninsula even before the outset of Korea's colonization in 1910. Rather, it was Manchuria's large-scale public projects that appealed to established investors like the old zaibatsu; Korea had remained a niche market for relatively new companies, such as Nitchitsu. Kang Jae Eun, a scholar of modern Korean social thought, attests that the new zaibatsu "earned substantial profits from investment in Korea in the pre-1930 period, and this created a basis for its growth thereafter."[39] This point is further explained by Soon Won Park: "industrial investment slackened in the 1920s until it again picked up in the early 1930s," thanks to new entrepreneurs, such as "the aggressive and ambitious Noguchi [Shitagau] of the newly emerging [Nitchitsu], a Japanese zaibatsu, boldly ventured into the then high-tech hydroelectric-chemical and textile industries in the colony's northern provinces and in the Seoul/In-ch'on industrial region."[40]

Moore provides a further historical explanation for Noguchi's success, which he believes derived inadvertently from a policy created by the governor-general of Korea. Responding to Japan's rice riots in 1918, the governor-general of Korea launched the "Program to Increase Rice Production" to secure the rice harvest in Korea—not in order to feed people in Korea but to send this staple food to Japan. For this purpose, the governor-general encouraged Korean farmers to use fertilizer to increase their yields. This policy gave an advantage to Noguchi's business in Korea, for the Nitchitsu factories in Japan had recently succeeded in using surplus electricity from the Sogi hydropower plant to synthesize low-cost ammonia to be used in fertilizer.[41] In 1925, with Morita Kazuo, an engineer and a classmate from Tokyo Imperial University, Noguchi established Chōsen Suiden Kabushikikaisha, a hydroelectric power company in Hŭngnam, in present-day North Korea.

Eventually, the Korean Peninsula drew attention as a potential field for investments, and as the competition in Korea became intense, projects grew in scale. According to Moore, Nitchitsu's unprecedented 700,000-kilowatt Sup'ung Dam project set it apart from other conglomerates both within and beyond Japan. At the same time, the governor-general of Korea was promoting Korean industrialization to serve the Japanese empire's wartime economic system.[42] The governor-general ardently supported Japanese businesses in Korea, even as he sought to avoid political turmoil on the peninsula. Bringing several conglomerates into competition with each other, the governor-general sought to ensure affordable electric power for households in Korea—a strategy deriving not from sympathy toward colonized subjects in Korea, but from his objective to maintain order by suppressing dissatisfaction with Japanese colonial expansionism.

According to the estimates of Kayashima Hidenobu, an engineer at Nitchitsu, the total amount of electric power generated at Nitchitsu's hydroelectric power stations in Korea amounted to 12 billion kilowatts per hour, close to the 12.2 billion produced at that time by the Tennessee Valley

Authority (TVA), a massive federal corporation in the United States.[43] And much as the TVA was established not merely to save the American economy after the Great Depression but also to channel new technology into military use,[44] Nitchitsu's technology was used to turn Korea into an "'advance military supply base' (*zenshin heitan kichi*) for Japan's penetration of China."[45]

During the last decade of the colonial period, Japan's deep involvement in the war was reflected in its investment in armaments and military manufacturing, such as textiles for uniforms, metals for machines, and chemicals for weaponry.[46] Historian of modern Korea, Kasuya Ken'ichi observes that Japanese big business groups and the colonial government were close partners in the financing, marketing, and administrative matters of these war-related, large-scale industries.[47] The success of his enterprise in the Korean Peninsula gave Noguchi confidence to expand his energy business into Manchuria. After World War I, the increasing demand for, and dearth of, petroleum as an energy source in Japan was obvious. Responding to this issue, Noguchi and others began researching the production of chemically synthesized oil. In 1940, a coal liquefaction factory of the South Manchuria Railway in Bujun (Fushun)[48] succeeded in producing (low-quality) synthetic oil from coal.[49] Nitchitsu followed suit, investing in a synthetic oil company in Kitsurin (Jilin) in 1942.[50] By this time, Noguchi had retired from business, having suffered from a cerebral hemorrhage in 1940, but his vision was shared and advanced by the rest of the company. By 1940, Nitchitsu's expansion reached its zenith, ranging from the northern part of the Korean Peninsula, which also produced synthetic oil, to Taiyuan in Shanxi Province, Taiwan, Hainan Island, Java, Sumatra, and Malaya. Among those overseas factories, Kōnan (Hŭngnam in present-day North Korea) was perhaps the biggest, with its company-owned housing complex being larger than the complex in Minamata.[51]

Upon Japan's defeat in World War II in 1945, all of Nitchitsu's properties and assets in these colonial lands were confiscated. Noguchi did not survive to witness this turn, as he had died the previous year. Although his death did not halt the expansion of his business empire, its operation was halted with the dissolution of the Japanese empire. Surprisingly, however, the factory in Minamata resumed its operation only two months after the end of the war. The severe food shortage meant that fertilizers were once again in high demand.

While Minamata factory experienced a swift return to operations, Nitchitsu as a zaibatsu failed to uphold itself even before the 1950's Enterprise Reorganization Act disbanded Nitchitsu officially. The act, implemented by the Supreme Commander of the Allied Powers (SCAP) in postwar occupied Japan, was intended to disempower zaibatsu and to distribute wealth more widely, thereby meeting the needs of the masses and helping them realize democracy. This was also the year when the Korean War broke out, and the SCAP was quite concerned about communist influences in Japan. To protect the capitalists in Japan, the SCAP allowed the former new zaibatsu to regroup. As a result, Nitchitsu became *Shin Nihon Chisso hiryō kabushiki-gaisha*, now referred to simply as Chisso.

CHISSO WORKERS AND MINAMATA FISHERS

Prior to 1945, when many Japanese people crossed the sea and channels to the empire's colonies in Taiwan, the Korean Peninsula, and Manchuria in search of employment opportunities, a number of Minamata residents migrated, too, finding work at various Nitchitsu sites. A book compiled by Matsuzaki Tsuguo and Okamoto Tatsuaki informs us of the experiences of these people. Okamoto worked for Chisso, served as the leader of the first union at the Minamata factory, and, together with Matsuzaki, collected volumes of oral history. One volume introduces the stories of those who returned from the colonial lands.

The book provides a gripping historical account of Japanese citizens' cruel treatment of the local laborers and the tensions between not only Japanese colonizers and Korean employees but also Korean workers and Chinese coolies. This part of history was not a memory that the returnees publicly embraced; one of the repatriates tells the editors that their time in Korea was something that they did not want to voluntarily reveal: "[After the war], associations for former soldiers and alumni associations for schools were organized everywhere, but, despite the fact that so many of us crossed the strait to go to Korea, no one suggested forming a group of returnees from Korea."[52] Even though Chisso and their workers detached themselves from their colonial history, Okamoto, in the epilogue to the volume, discloses the fact that upon their return, the leaders of Nitchitsu in Korea assumed the administrative positions and management offices of Chisso's Minamata factory.[53]

The first part of the comprehensive six-volume work by Okamoto demonstrates that the modern system sharpened the divisions in the existing hierarchy in Minamata. Timothy S. George describes Minamata's existing social order: "The replacement of the old samurai and landlord families by a large modern corporation did not make Minamata society any less hierarchical. If anything, it strengthened the hierarchy, widened the gap between top and bottom, and intensified the discrimination and prejudice against those on the lower rungs."[54]

Drawing upon Okamoto's collection of oral histories, I want to articulate a perspective and worldview shared by former Chisso employees, especially the repatriates, better to understand the discriminatory treatment of Minamata disease sufferers, which will be further examined in the following chapters.

Turning to these oral testimonies will reveal, on the one hand, that Minamata disease did not *create* a division between the Chisso workers and Minamata sufferers but rather *intensified* a preexisting division. On the other hand, the disease did create a divide among the fishers, as we will see in chapter 3. In this regard, Okamoto's detailed study, which focuses on the three communities of Tsukinoura, Dezuki (sometimes pronounced Detsuki), and Yudō in Minamata, is especially relevant, as sixty percent of certified Minamata patients between 1956 and 1957 were from these communities.[55]

We may begin with Nakayama Miyo, of Dezuki, who lived in Shanghai as a family member of a Chisso employee. Nakayama testifies that upon returning from the colonized land, she had no difficulties in making friends: "Back then, one out of three Dezuki households was *kaisha-iki*, or Chisso employees. That many people depended on kaisha, or the company [referring to Chisso]."[56] Nakayama's friends included the Fukumitsu and Miyoshi families, who had also returned from the colonies; the Fukumitsu family returned from Hŭngnam in Korea, and the Miyoshi family from Manchuria. Nakayama was proud that her husband worked for Chisso and refused to be friends with women, or oyster harvesters, or whose husbands were mere fishers because they would do nothing but "chatter."[57]

Her testimony reveals that even in the areas with a high concentration of certified Minamata patients, working for Chisso was embraced as an integral part of one's individual and family identity, signifying a high social status that often bore with it a correspondingly contemptuous attitude toward non-Chisso employees. Such pride prevented those affiliated with Chisso from interacting with fishers. This psychological distance from the fishers only intensified after Minamata disease was initially observed among the fishers and their families. Discrimination against the sufferers did not arise solely out of misconception of the disease being contagious; rather, some repatriates found in the disease justification for their poor treatment of the fishers afflicted with the disease.

Minamata fishers were in fact more than simply "oyster harvesters." The many ways in which they gathered food in and along the Shiranui Sea of Minamata points to the rich biodiversity of the area. Some gathered seaweed and seashells at the beach, while others used fishing rods and bait to catch fish in the Shiranui Sea. Still, others worked together to operate fishing boats, casting nets and harpooning. Some fishers caught octopus, while others also grew vegetables in fields in their spare time. As Chisso flourished and expanded, more employees were hired and came to live in Minamata, thus increasing the demand for fish. And as the population of Minamata grew, so did the number of fishers, many of whom came from the Amakusa Islands, on the other side of the Shiranui Sea.

The discriminatory attitude toward these fishers on the part of individual Chisso employees could also be observed in the company's collective treatment of the fishers. In 1926, the Chisso factory in Minamata had begun a large-scale operation to produce synthetic ammonium sulfate for fertilizer. Its financial success elevated Chisso to the position of the top fertilizer company in Japan. In this process, however, the factory spawned *kurodobe*, or black mud, which was released into the Shiranui Sea. This black mud suffocated seaweed and shellfish by the seashore, resulting in poor harvests for fishers. *Minamata gyogyō kumiai* (the Minamata Fishing Cooperative), having received complaints from the fishers, negotiated with Chisso for compensation. Not well prepared to contend with a rising corporation, the cooperative's negotiations with the corporation resulted in favor of Chisso: the fishers received money, but the company offered it not as "compensation" but as a one-time "donation," allowing Chisso to avoid admission of any wrongdoing. The agreement that was reached between the fishers and then Nitchitsu stated that the cooperative would never again bring this issue to the company.[58] Thus, it was not only Chisso that disregarded the fishers' claims but the cooperative itself that failed to recognize the magnitude of the negotiations, resulting in jeopardized livelihoods. Thirty years later, when the "mysterious disease" was widely observed among first cats and then people, Chisso was the last to be blamed, due in part to this historical background.

The Miyoshi family lived in Dezuki, where by 1955 one-third of the households had at least one Chisso employee.[59] Miyoshi Masahiro recalls that "the lives of Chisso workers and those of non-Chisso workers were quite different. Girls wanted to marry a Chisso employee, even if he was lame or physically handicapped, because of his steady income.[60] Chisso workers had cash. They were well off in Dezuki. By contrast, non-Chisso workers had no secure means of income (and thus were not preferred as marriage partners)."[61] Chisso workers with steady paychecks were highly appealing as ideal husbands to young women. "The first is Chisso workers, the last is fishers" was the saying in Dezuki regarding the choice of one's spouse. In addition, in the Dezuki community, fishers were relative newcomers, which made it difficult for them to earn respect.[62] Miyoshi's statement illustrates the disparate positions that Chisso workers and fishers occupied in the community's socioeconomic hierarchy.

Although the Chisso workers generally looked down on fishers, the factory employees took pride in their ostensibly progressive political views. Most employees were aware of workers' rights. Overall, they were educated on matters of labor, studying the conditions of workers and alert to unjust social structures. When it came to politics, then, the fishers were more inclined to vote for members of the conservative party, while Chisso workers tended to vote for more progressive candidates.

Nakayama Miyo, a repatriate from Shanghai, recalls the election season when the division between Chisso employees and fishers became more apparent: "Minamata was always heated around the time of the election, and Dezuki was one of the [most heated] communities. Chisso workers were reformists, called *kakushin-kei* (the progressives), and supporters of the Social Democratic Party of Japan while farmers and fishers backed the Liberal Democratic Party (LDP), a conservative leading party. We were clearly split."[63] Thus, notwithstanding their progressive vision, many Chisso workers paid little attention to the sufferings of the fishers. Manchurian returneee Miyoshi Chiyoka explains why many low-income farmers and fishers supported the LDP: the party would bribe farmers and fishers, in particular those with unstable incomes or otherwise in need of cash.[64] Whether Miyoshi's speculation was accurate, her statement indicates the Chisso workers' self-righteous position. They perceived themselves as claiming the moral high ground, for their votes could not be bought—a self-perception indicating disdain for those who allegedly accepted money in return for votes.

But even Chisso employees, though taking pride in working for the company, were not always aligned politically with their employer. For example, in Minamata's first mayoral election in 1950 (Minamata was incorporated as a city in 1949), Hashimoto Hikoshichi, a former Chisso factory manager, campaigned for the mayorship. He won the election thanks to support from his fellow factory workers, even as Chisso executives, most of whom had returned from one of the largest Hŭngnam factories in Korea and had looked down upon the Minamata factory as a small countryside operation, did not endorse Hashimoto.[65] Thus, Chisso factory workers, though perceiving themselves as socially elevated, were aware of the fragility of their status.

According to sociologist Irokawa Daikichi, who headed *Shiranui kai sōgō gakujutsu chōsadan* (an interdisciplinary investigating team of the Shiranui Sea from 1976–1981),[66] this fragility was the product of Chisso's strategic reproduction of the social hierarchy in postwar Minamata so as to maintain its hegemony. Chisso hired white-collar, full-time employees with higher degrees from technical colleges and universities outside Minamata, while Minamata locals were hired as unskilled workers, some of whom were low-paid day laborers. To secure the social order which favored it, Chisso prevented Minamata from building any institutions of higher education, thus allowing the corporation to continue its exploitation of the people in Minamata, who became its "willing" hostages.[67]

REBELLIONS BY MINAMATA FISHERS AND CHISSO EMPLOYEES

As early as the 1950s, Minamata residents took notice of strange behavior among the cats in their village. Some wandered endlessly in circles, while others, moving erratically into the sea, drowned. It was not long before people in Minamata began experiencing numbness in their limbs or uncontrollable tremors over their entire bodies, leading to death. After many human and nonhuman lives succumbed to such agonizing deaths, in 1955, a medical team from Kumamoto University admitted that these symptoms signaled a "mysterious disease" that was neither contagious nor confined to fishers but was the result of neurological damage that cut across professional and economic divides. In the following year, the team announced that the illness was possibly being caused by Chisso's wastewater. Nonetheless, Chisso, in tandem with Japan's Ministry of International Trade and Industry, dismissed the medical experts' public statement and continued to release contaminated water, despite the Minamata Fishing Cooperative's request to halt its release. By 1959, the research accomplished by the medical team revealed the culprit: methylmercury found in Chisso's wastewater was the cause of the illness.

As knowledge of the illness and its cause spread beyond Minamata, sales of fresh fish plummeted, to the particular detriment of fishers and fishmongers. On August 6, 1959, 400 members from the cooperative and the *Sengyo Nakagaishō Kumiai* (Fish Broker Association) demonstrated at the Chisso factory, asking for 100 million yen as compensation for their lost business. When negotiations with Chisso failed to produce the desired payout, the fishers flooded into the factory and arrested its managers. With the aim of settling the dispute, Kumamoto Governor Teramoto Kōsaku organized a group to discuss the issue. The eventual "resolution" afforded little help to the fishers. On October 17, 1959, in a show of solidarity, fishers from the Fishers Cooperative, comprising regional members from the regions of Uto, Shimomashiki, Yashiro, Taura, Ashikita, Amakusa, arrived in sixty boats to plea with Chisso to stop the discharge of the water.[68]

But enjoying support from citizens, politicians, and the wider business world, Chisso declined to negotiate with the fishers. Growing impatient in the wake of failed attempts in August and October to reach an agreement, approximately 2,000 fishers forced their way into the factory on November 2, clashing with the police force guarding the factory. Over 100 people were injured in the confrontation.[69] Notwithstanding the conflicts and the fishers' pleas, fifty representatives of twenty-eight organizations in Minamata and its vicinity—from political affiliations, business organizations, and labor unions—requested that Governor Teramoto Kōsaku to secure Chisso's operation, allowing it to continue discharging the wastewater.[70]

Newspapers at this time reported that Minamata citizens were more concerned with preserving the tax income from Chisso, which constituted more than half of the city's revenue, than they were with addressing and alleviating the fishers' sufferings. The newspapers, instead of questioning the prioritization of the corporation's health over the health of humans and the environment, noted that even a short-term halt in Chisso's operation would affect the lives of 50,000 Minamata citizens one way or another.[71]

An informative essay by Ding Weiwei cites a 1959 newspaper article condoning the prioritization of livelihood over lives: "Over 57% of the city's entire revenue, which equated to 1.9 billion yen, came from Chisso's property tax and the Chisso employees' municipal tax. The 3,600 Chisso employees numbered twelve times more than the member of the Fishing Cooperative."[72] Repeatedly observed, the city's collective attitude was not one of sympathy toward Minamata sufferers but rather one of adamancy for the protection of Chisso. Eventually, however, some Chisso workers began to see themselves not as victims whose jobs were made vulnerable by fishers blaming the company for their disease, but rather as victimizers, complicit with Chisso in allowing the factory to continue destroying people's lives as well as the environment.

In 1968, when Chisso finally stopped releasing methylmercury, the company's union workers had to face the wrongdoings wrought by the corporation, admitting that they were accountable for Minamata disease.[73] Former Chisso worker, union member, and author of *Minamata byō to rōdōsha* (Minamata disease and workers) Ishida Hirofumi confessed that the labor union for too long regarded itself as a victim because the sufferers' accusation of Chisso was used to suppress the workers' wages. With profound regret for their neglect of the plight of the fishers, the Chisso labor union publicly issued *Haji sengen,* or a declaration of shame, in its newsletter *Sairen* (Siren) in 1968. In this declaration, the workers reflected critically on their neglect and admitted that they had dismissed the pains of the Minamata sufferers, despite the fact that Chisso, their employer, had inflicted suffering on the fishers as well as their families and friends.[74]

Throughout the tumultuous decade of the 1950s, the union demanded that Chisso and the Kumamoto prefectural government uncover the cause of the "strange disease,"[75] even as it insisted that the factory should not be shut down. Union leader Yamashita Yoshihiro was a leading figure working on behalf of Minamata sufferers. Born in Hamgyŏngnam, Korea, under Japanese colonization, Yamashita and his family were among those who repatriated to Japan. Known by his nickname Zenkan-san, he was trusted and relied upon by the sufferers.[76] In an interview, Yamashita recalled his time at Chisso: "The union gave tents to the fishers and Minamata sufferers who came to the factory for the sit-in. But the company disapproved this action, and took the tents away. Moreover, the union did not unanimously side with sufferers, who demanded the factory be closed, which would endanger the union members' livelihood."[77] Although Yamashita showed sympathy to those fishers, he admitted that politically he was still on the side of the company.[78]

This chapter has outlined Chisso's history, its role in the modernization of Japan, and the Minamata people's embrace of Chisso's expansion and the social order that came with it. I have examined the life of Chisso's founder, Noguchi Shitagau, Chisso's expansion to colonial lands, and the Chisso workers' complex relations to fishers. As we observed in chapter 1, modern society presupposes that humans are independent and autonomous agents, exercising free will in making decisions. This concept of personhood is also based on the presupposition that humans are rational agents. Thus conceived, humans are not only divided from nonhumans and other-than-humans: in the end, each individual has to bear responsibility for her decisions, with poor choices being attributed to the failure of rational thinking. One can blame none other than oneself.

The problem with this conception of selfhood does not lie in its underlying myth of autonomy, but rather in its application. This fiction of autonomy, as we saw in chapter 1, produces and maintains a system of precarity, severing humans from fellow humans, nonhumans, and other-than-humans. But reconfiguring the ontological story we tell ourselves may offer possibilities for recognizing and redressing such precarity in a manner that would foster the protection of human life and the natural environment.

This modern condition of separation from one another and from the natural environment may be seen as one mode of what Max Weber called "disenchantment."[79] But the characterization of modern society as disenchanted has been challenged by many scholars. Jason Ā. Josephson-Storm, for example, claims that the modern world remains enchanted, pointing to the fact today we remain fascinated with occultism and witchcraft, and allured by paranormal phenomena.[80] Although I agree that attraction to such things has never disappeared, the occult, witchcraft, and paranormal phenomena have been excluded from the public realm for a long time, relegated to the marginal, including in academia.[81]

The history of the study of religion in Japan bears out this point. Inoue Enryō, who studies Buddhism in its encounter with Western modernity, has attempted to conceive of Buddhism in a manner that makes it compatible with the Western notion of "religion." Protecting Buddhism from accusations of superstition and ensuring Buddhism, Inoue reconceptualizes Buddhism so as to find acceptance as a "rational" religion in the eyes of Westerners. If we think that modern society is not entirely disenchanted and that reenchantment is crucial, we perhaps need to re-constellate our worldviews, retrieving the "irrational" from the peripheral to examine.

To this end, I take the reimagination of the modern "person" as a rational, independent, and autonomous agent, to be urgent. Jane Bennett's approach to "enchantment" offers a helpful start for this undertaking. Bennett defines "enchantment" as "a state of openness to the disturbing-captivating elements in everyday experience" that is "operative in a world without telos."[82] She elaborates further, describing enchantment as "a feeling of being connected in an affirmative way to existence." The stories in the following chapters, where we examine the lives and thoughts of Hongan no kai's members, will bear out and extend Bennett's theoretical insights with lived experiences, suggesting a way of reconceiving personhood and enchanting existence.

Because Bennett has argued that "enchantment is a mood with ethical potential,"[83] the ontological and epistemological shifts that would attend enchantment adumbrate an ethical project:

> I pursue an ethics that applies to cross-species as well as interhuman relations. I first broaden the sense of what agency means to cover the ability to make a difference in the world without knowing exactly what you are doing, and I project this agency as distributed, to varying degrees, to atoms that move, plants that engage their environment, and animals that communicate, as well as humans that write onto-stories, protest war, engage in hate speech, and so forth.[84]

As we will see, Bennett's remarks resonate with Hongan no kai's praxes, which contribute to ethical discourse in general with their reconfigurations of ontology and epistemology, but also particularly to environmental ethics, providing a new worldview—the world janaka shaba, or a world otherwise—where agency is assigned not to individuals but assemblages.

In addressing the ideas and actions of Hongan no kai, I do not intend to offer an uncritical picture that portrays their various endeavors as uniformly successful. Nonetheless, I find it worthwhile to investigate them at a time when our supposedly rational undertakings have led to the destruction of lives and livelihoods. In the next four chapters, I consider three individual members of Hongan no kai: Sugimoto Eiko, Ogata Masato, and Ishimure Michiko. Tracing their life stories and lived experiences will help delineate their vision of a world otherwise that may offer, as Bennett puts it, "disturbing" elements but may thereby provide a perspective for reconceiving ourselves and our surroundings.

NOTES

1. Timothy S. George, *Minamata: Pollution and the Struggle for Democracy in Postwar Japan* (Cambridge, MA: Harvard University Asia Center, 2001).
2. Ishimure, Michiko, *Soseishita tamshii o nosete* (On board with the resurrected spirits) (Tokyo: Kawadeshobō shinsha, 2013, 96.
3. Livia Monnet, "'Another World in This World': Slow Violence, Environmental Time, and the Decolonial Imagination in Ishimure Michiko's *Villages of*

the Gods," in *Ishimure Michiko's Writing in Ecocritical Perspective: Between Sea and Sky*, eds. by Bruce Allen and Yuki Masami (Lanham, MD: Lexington Books, 2015), 151.

4. Historian Carol Gluck defines modernity not as a "trope, theory, project, or destination" but as a "condition." Carol Gluck, "The End of Elsewhere: Writing Modernity Now," *The American Historical Review*, 116, no. 3 (2011): 676. Aslo, the following two scholars are helpful to ponder the concept of modernity with respect to that of nature: "Japan's [modernity] was not a deformed modernity or a belated modernity, but a rue modernity with all the problems that arise from it. In order to understand this global process, we must ask what makes some modernities more productive of justice in public life and others less so. Differing concepts of nature are part of the answer." Julia Adeney Thomas, *Reconfiguring Modernity: Concepts of Nature in Japanese Political Ideology* (Berkeley, CA: University of California Press, 2002), 29; and "Oddly, this 'ecological modernization' theory sounds similar to that modernization ditty crooned by Fukuzawa Yukichi and Maruyama Masao decades earlier: modernity, no matter its form, always preaches triumph over, or 'disengagement' from, nature." Brett L. Walker, *Toxic Archipelago: A History of Industrial Disease in Japan* (Seattle, WA: University of Washington Press, 2011), 215.

5. Ogata, Masato, "*Hongan no kai* zadankai: tsukamidokoro no nai bakemono" (*Hongan no kai* discussion: Unfathomable phantom), *Tamashii utsure* 41 (2010): 27.

6. Dominic Boyer, "Anthropology Electric," *Cultural Anthropology* 30, no. 4 (2015): 532.

7. According to Yoshimi, *Electrical Review*—a weekly magazine specializing in electrical engineering—was first published in 1883 and was followed by several more of its kind: *Electrical World, American Electrician, Electrical Engineering, Western Electrician,* and *Scientific American.* Yoshimi, Shun'ya, *"Koe" no shihonshugi* (Voice and Capitalism) (Tokyo: Kōdansha, 1995), 59. The readership of *Electrical World,* reports that Yoshimi amounted to 17,000 by the year 1895, indicating the emergence of a new industry together with a new occupational class. Yoshimi takes note that these magazines displayed uninhibitedly discriminatory views toward African Americans, native Americans, farmers, and women, from which we can deduce that Caucasian males may have dominated this new class of electricians. Yoshimi, *"Koe" no shihonshugi*, 61–62.

8. One such movement was the *Jiyū Minken Undō* (Movement for Liberty and People's Rights) organized by the former warrior class of the samurai. Medical journalist Hiroko Aihara gave a presentation on the overlap between the areas where the movement arose and the facilities that the government established after the Fukushima nuclear reactor meltdown. Hiroko Aihara, "Investigation of the Global Hibakusha and the Role of the Information Center," May 28, 2017, at *Genpatsu saigai jōhō senta,* Fukushima.

9. A theological explanation for electricity is found in a fascinating chapter by Brett Malcolm Grainger, *Church in the Wild: Evangelicals in Antebellum America* (Cambridge, MA: Harvard University Press, 2019), 168–169. In Japan, Akashi Hirotaka advocated "denki Shinto" or "Electric Shinto" in which Akashi explains

the power of Shinto divinity by the function of electricity. Tanaka, Satoshi, *Kaibutsu kagakusha no jidai* (The era of monsterous scientists) (Tokyo: Shōbunsha, 1998), 35–52.

10. Tanaka, Satoshi, *Kenkou hō to iyashi no shakaishi* (Sociological history of staying healthy and healing) (Tokyo: Seikyūsha, 2006), 99. Ginoza, Naomi, *Modan raifu to sensou—sukurīn no naka no joseitachi* (Modern life and war—women on the screen) (Tokyo: Yoshikawa koubunkan, 2013), 32–33. The term *bunka seikatsu* was coined by Morimoto Koukichi, then a professor at Hokkaido University. Tanaka, Satoshi, *Denki wa dare no monoka* (To whom electricity belongs) (Tokyo: Shōbunsha, 2015), 82.

11. The influential politician Gotō Shinpei, for example, advocated the use of electricity and home appliances by heading a group called *Katei denki fukyū kyōkai* (Cooperative for Popularizing Domestic Electric Appliances), staging the Electricity Expo, organizing public lectures, and publishing magazines. Tanaka, *Denki wa dare no monoka,* 82–83. The fervor for electric power at the time culminated in 1922 when the renowned electric engineer Yamamoto Tadaoki had built his home in Mejiro, Tokyo, which was fully equipped with electrical power. His Spanish-style house represented culture, civilization, and a civilized lifestyle through the use of electricity. Tanaka, *Denki wa dare no monoka,* 85.

12. Tanaka also reports a case of Namerikawa town, in Toyama, a small fishing village known for the origin of a rice riot (*kome soudou*), was also the birthplace of *dentō sōgi*, an uprising over electricity rights. Namerikawa villagers stood up against an electric company that monopolized the market and tried to raise the price of electricity. Tanaka, *Denki wa dare no monoka,* 171–172. The cases of riots and conflicts eventually dwindled down because the number of electric companies rose to 810 by 1926, which made the monopolization of the market harder.

13. In 1925, when a battle between two construction companies broke out over a newly established electric power company in Tsurumi, near Tokyo, a plan to construct a new electric power plant was the cause of this battle, which would support the restoration of the Tokyo metropolitan area after the Great Kantō Earthquake of 1923. The subcontractors' workers physically attacked one another, resulting in over 500 arrests. For more details, see Aoyama, Kōji, *Tatakai no kouzu* (The structure of the battle), vols. 1 and 2 (Tokyo: Asahi shimbunsha, 1991).

14. Tanaka, *Denki wa dare no monoka,* 7.

15. Noguchi himself preferred to be called Jun or Juntarō, another pronunciation for the Chinese character of *Shitagau*, here resenting this uncommon name; however, I will use his birth name, Shitagau.

16. Barbara Molony, *Technology and Investment: The Prewar Japanese Chemical Industry* (Cambridge, MA: Harvard University Press, 1990), 63.

17. Molony, *Technology and Investment,* 63. Also, Oshio Takeshi, "Reimeiki kābaido bijinesu no keifu to Noguchi Jun—Sankyozawa kābaido seizōsho kara Nihon Chisso Hiryō ni itaru michisuji" (the Dawn of Carbide business in Japan and Jun Noguchi) *The Papers and Proceedings of Economics,* 153 (2017), especially 148, note 9.

18. Oshio, "reimeiki kābaido bijinesu," 135.

19. Molony, *Technology and Investment,* 63.

20. Molony, *Technology and Investment,* 63.

21. Noguchi's interests in carbide is detailed by Oshio's "Reimeiki kābaido business." Notes 34–43, 151–152.

22. Other chemicals included ammonia, explosives, acetylene, acetic acid vinyl, butanol, esters, acetates. Molony, *Technology and Investment,* 66.

23. According to Chisso's history book, *Fūsetsu no hyakunen: Chisso kabushikikaisha shi* (A hundred years of hardships: history of Chisso corporation), Noguchi was involved with the establishment of Sogi electric company in the summer and fall of 1905, Oshio, based upon the official document, asserts that his involvement began already in 1904. Oshio, "Reimeiki kābaido bijinesu," 141–142.

24. Molony, *Technology and Investment,* 67, 69.

25. Molony, *Technology and Investment,* 70. Oshio, "Reimeiki kābaido bijinesu,"

26. George, *Minamata,* 17.

27. Kobayashi, Naoki, "Sousetsu: 'Minamata' no gensetsuteki kouchiku" (Summary: Construction of Minamata discourse), in *Minamata no gensetsu to hyōshō* (Minamata discourse and symbolism), ed. Kobayashi Naoki (Tokyo: Fujiwara shoten, 2007), 17.

28. Molony, *Technology and Investment,* 71. According to Odagiri and Gotō, the scale of this power plant was 800 kilowatts. Hiroyuki Odagiri and Akira Gotō, *Technology and Industrial Development in Japan: Building Capabilities by Learning, Innovation and Public Policy* (Oxford: Clarendon Press, 1996), 77.

29. In 1906, a year before Noguchi established his Minamata company, he had heard news that two Germans, "A. Frank and N. Caro, [had] invented a new method to produce calcium cyanamide to be used as fertilizer." Odagiri and Gotō, *Technology and Industrial Development in Japan,* 77. Always keen on new technology, Noguchi decided to sail to Germany, accompanied by the co-owner, Fujiyama, to obtain the patent right for the method. The negotiation was full of challenges because Noguchi was bidding against representatives of already established Japanese zaibatsu, or conglomerates, such as Masuda Takashi of Mitsui and Hara Takashi (also known as Hara Kei, who later became the prime minister of Japan) of Furukawa. However, Noguchi's enthusiasm and connections from Siemens allowed him to win the patent right over the zaibatsu. Molony, *Technology and Investment,* 73.

30. Molony, *Technology and Investment,* 86.

31. Okamoto, Tatsuaki, *Minamatabyō no minshūshi* (People's history of Minamata disease), vol. 1, *Mae no jidai—butai to shite no mittsu no mura to Minamata wan* (Pre-disease: Three villages and Minamata [Shiranui] Bay as a cradle of disease) (Tokyo: Nihon hyōronsha, 2015), 7.

32. George, *Minamata,* 18.

33. George, *Minamata,* 20.

34. Kamoi Yū, *Noguchi Shitagau: Ningen to jigyō* (Noguchi Shitagau: His personality and business) (Tokyo: Tōkōsha, 1943), 157. Kamoi praises Noguchi's dedication to the company, informing readers that Noguchi sometimes worked until

two in the morning and occasionally stayed overnight at the factory. Also see Kamoi, *Noguchi Shitagau,* 218.

35. In a book review on Moore, Juergen P. Melzer criticizes Moore's avoidance of treating figures such as Noguchi as well as other new zaibatsu leaders. Juergen P. Melzer, "Review: Constructing East Asia: Technology, Ideology, and Empire in Japan's Wartime Era, 1931–1945," *Japan Review* 27 (2014): 244.

36. Fukai, Jun'ichi, *Minamatabyō no seijikeizaigaku: Sangyōshiteki haikei to gyousei sekinin,* (Tokyo: Keisō shobō, 1999), 1.

37. Michiko, *Sosei shita tamashii o nosete,* 19.

38. Kamoi, *Noguchi Shitagau,* 219.

39. Kan, Chae-On, *Chosen ni okeru Nitchitsu kontserun* (The Japan nitrogen group in Korea) (Tokyo: Fuji shuppan, 1985).

40. Soon Won Park, "The First Generation of Korean Skilled Workers: the Onoda Cement Sŭunghori Factory," *The Journal of Korean Studies* 7 (1990): 59.

41. Aaron Stephen Moore, *Constructing East Asia: Technology, Ideology, and Empire in Japan's Wartime Era, 1931–1945* (Stanford, CA: Stanford University Press, 2013), 153.

42. Moore, *Constructing East Asia,* 154–155.

43. Kayashima, Hidenobu, "Fusenkō hatsuden kouji to Kōnan koujou no kensetsu" (Construction of the electronic station at Puch'ŏn-gang and a factory at Hŭngnam), in *Kikigaki Minamata Minshūshi,* vol. 5, *Shokuminchi wa tengoku datta* (Oral history of Minamata people, vol. 5, The colony was the heaven), eds. by Okamoto Tatasuaki and Matsuzaki Tsuguo (Tokyo: Sōfūkan, 1997 [1990]), 35.

44. Fukai, *Minamatabyō no seijikeizaigaku,* 1.

45. Carter J. Eckert, *Offspring of Empire: The Koch'ang Kims and the Colonial Origins of Korean Capitalism, 1876–1945* (Seattle, WA: University of Washington Press, 2014), 114.

46. Park, "The First Generation of Korean Skilled Workers," 59–60.

47. Kasuya, Ken'ichi, "Senji keizai to Chōsen ni okeru nitchitsu zaibatsu no tenkai" (The development of the new zaibatsu and the wartime economy), in *Chōsenshi kenkyūkai Ronbunshū,* 12 (1975): 175–209. Another example was Tōyō Bōseki, or the Toyo Spinning Company. In the 1930s, its branch factories in Korea yielded large profits because local wages were lower and no legal restrictions on working hours existed. Tōyō Bōseki, ed., *Tōyō Bōseki 70-nen shi* (Osaka: Tōyō Bōseki, 1953), 377–379. These profits sustained the firm while the home factories performed badly. Also see Mistuhiko Kimura, "The Economics of Japanese Imperialism in Korea, 1910–1939," *Economic History Review, New Series* 48, no. 3 (1995): 564.

48. The South Manchuria Railway was Japanese empire's policy company overseeing the railways in northeast of China, established in 1906, after Japan took over the area from Russia subsequent to the Russo-Japan War.

49. Mine, Takeshi, "'Manshū' kagaku kougyou no kaihatsu to shin Chūgoku e no keishou" (The development of chemical factories in Manchuria and the transformation to the new China), *Ajia kenkyū* 52, no. 1 (2006): 37 and note 12. It was not until 1944 that the factory produced synthetic oil although only the small amount of 4,310 tons, which was used for airplanes and automobiles.

50. Mine, "Manshū' kagaku kougyou no kaihatsu," 25, 27.

51. See Tsujihara, Makihiko, "Chōsen Chisso Hiryō no Kōnan chiku shataku gai nit suite: Noguchi kenkyūsho shozou shiryou o mochiite" (Restoration of the Company Town Plan Constructed by the Chōsen Chisso Hiryō Hungnam Factory: Using Materials Owned by the Noguchi Institute), *Nihon kenchiku gakkai keikakukei ronbunshū* 77, no. 671 (2012): 135–142.

52. Okamoto, *Minamatabyō no minshūshi,* 317.

53. Okamoto, Tatsuaki, "*Atogaki*" (Epilogue), in *Kikigaki Minamata Minshūshi,* ed. Okamoto Tatasuaki and Matsuzaki Tsuguo, (Tokyo: Sōfūkan, 1997 [1990]), 345. Also, one of the Chisso workers, Fuchigami Kazuyoshi, testified that those who returned from the Korean Peninsula were regarded highly, reflecting the commercial success in Korea. *NHK Rekishi shougen purojekuto: Nihonjin wan ani o mezashite kitanoka* (NHK Historical testimonies project: what did Japanese tried to achieve?) no. 2, *Minamata—Sengo fukkō kara kougai e* (Minamata—the Restoration of the war destruction to the public pollution), aired on July 13, 2013. The transcript is available at https://www2.nhk.or.jp/archives/shogenarchives/shogen/movie.cgi?das_id=D000 1130186_00000&seg_number=001. Furthermore, The continuation of the prewar system may remind one of the aftermath of the notorious Unit 731, which had conducted vivisection and cruel experiments on local prisoners (and possibly American POWs) in Manchuria during the war. Doctors and scientists who had been in this unit assumed important positions after the war in their own fields—leading the South Pole expedition as scientists or heading Midori jūji, one of the larger blood banks in Japan. See, for example, Sheldon H. Harris, *Factories of Death: Japanese Biological Warfare, 1932–1945, and the American Cover-up* (London: Routledge, 2002).

54. George, *Minamata*, 28. Also, centering on the Minamata castle, such social rungs were maintained concentrically, and the farther one lived from the center, the more intense the discriminatory gaze, was even before the emergence of Minamata disease. For more details, see Irokawa, Daikichi, *Minamata—sono sabetsu no fūdo to rekishi: Shiranuikai ichi chōsadan'in no shōgen* (Minamata—the history and environment of discrimination: A testimony of a member of Shiranui Sea Investigative Group) (Kumamoto: Hankougai Minamata kyōtōkaigi jimukyoku, 1980), 42–45.

55. Okamoto, *Minamatabyō no minshūshi,* 3. Okamoto adds that these three communities appear indistinct from each other as rural villages, but even in the 1970s, the Minamata people could tell which of the three a person came from by his or her appearance (mannerisms, dialect, and ambiance). Historically, the Tsukinoura community was the oldest, tracing its origin back to the Tokugawa era, and the villagers' livelihood depended primarily upon farming their land, not on fishing. Dezuki, on the other hand, was a relatively new community that came into being in the 1920s and early 1930s and largely consisted of Chisso employees who had originally migrated from the nearby island of Amakusa. According to Okamoto, there was no residential house in this community in the nineteenth century, and in the middle of 1920s, first forty households were established. Yudō was a mixture of old and new: it had had a small number of residents dating back to the Tokugawa era and newcomers after the Meiji, and most villagers were engaged in the fishery. Okamoto, *Minamatabyō no minshūshi,* 7 and 154. Also, see George, *Minamata,* 27–30.

56. Okamoto, *Minamatabyō no minshūshi,* 232.
57. Okamoto, *Minamatabyō no minshūshi,* 232.
58. Kobayashi, "Sousetsu: 'Minamata' no gensetsuteki kouchiku," 18–19. Also see Miyazawa Nobuo, *Minamatabyō jiken 40-nen* (Fukuoka: Ashi shobō, 1997).
59. Okamoto, *Minamatabyō no minshūshi*, 225.
60. This quote denigrates people with physical challenges, which does not reflect my own opinion.
61. Okamoto, *Minamatabyō no minshūshi*, 226–227.
62. Okamoto, *Minamatabyō no minshūshi*, 245.
63. Okamoto, *Minamatabyō no minshūshi*, 227.
64. Okamoto, *Minamatabyō no minshūshi*, 227.
65. Hashimoto served as a mayor for four terms until 1970, except for four years after the 1958 election when he lost the election to a rival who was supported by the corporation.
66. The historical and philosophical significance of the team's attempt has been studied by, for example, Morishita Naoki, "Minamatabyō shi ni okeru 'Shiranui kai sōgō gakujutsu chōsadan' no ichi—jinbun shakaikagaku kenkyū no 'kyōdō koui' ni tsuite" (Locating the 'Shiranui Sea Interdisciplinary Investigation Team' in the history of Minamata disease—on collaborative researches of humanities and social sciences) in *Seizongaku kenkyū sentā hōkoku* 14: *"Kotonari" no rikigaku—mainoritī o meguru kenkyū to houhou no jissenteki kadai* (Power dynamics of differences—practical problems of methodology in minority studies) eds. Yamamoto Takanori and Takahashi Shin'ichi: (2010): 319–348, and Komatsubara Orika, "'Kougai mondai' kara 'kankyō mondai' e: Minamata chiiki ni okeru 'Shiranui kai sōgō gakujutsu chōsadan' no katsudou o tegakari ni" (From the issue of "public pollution" to that of environment: with the study of "Shiranui Sea Interdisciplinary Investigation Team" in Minamata region) *Gendai seimei tetsugaku kenkyū* 7 (2018): 74–106.
67. Irokawa, *Minamata,* 46–48.
68. Shinmoto Masafumi, "Minamatabyō jiken ni okeru 'daisansha kikan' no mondai" *Kyushu Kyōritsu Daigaku Keizaigakubu Kiyō* 114 (2008): 2–3.
69. Takamine, *Minamata byō o shitteimasuka*, 14.
70. Shinmoto, "Minamatabyō jiken," 4.
71. Takamine, *Minamata byō o shitteimasuka*, 14. The newspaper is *Kumamoto Nichinichi Shimbun,* November 8, 1959.
72. Ding, Weiwei, "Fukushima genpatsu jiko to 'Minamata' gensetsu ni kansuru ichikousatsu: Kanrenshiryou no bunseki o rei ni" (A study of the Fukushima nuclear accident and the discourse on "Minamata": Analyzing the related documents), *Mediagaku: Bunka to komyunikēshon* 29 (2014): 91. The cited newspaper article is in *Nishinihon shimbun*, December 17, 1959.
73. The factory's labor union was formed in 1946 with 3,214 members, as informed by the *Nihon Chisso hiryō kabushikigaisha Minamata kōjō rōdō kumiai* (hereafter the Chisso Labor Union or the union). Resurrected after the Enterprise Reorganization Act in postwar Japan in 1950 as *Shin Nihon Chisso hiryō kabushikigaisha* (Shin-Nitchitsu, or New Nitchitsu, and after this year, I refer to it as Chisso). The workers started the new Progressive Labor Union with a membership of slightly

over 3,000. In 1953, the union went on strike and demanded the following three points: to redress the discriminatory treatment against low-ranking workers, to make a shift from a daily payment to a monthly salary, and to apply a retirement policy to every worker at 55 years of age, most of which the demands were accepted. Oishi Yutaka, "Sengo Nihon no shakaiundō ni okeru Chisso rōdōundō no ichizuke—mou hitotsu no Minamata" (Situating the Chisso labor movement in Japan's postwar social movements—Another face of Minamata), *Ohara shakai mondai kenkyūsho zasshi*, 630 (2011): 19.

74. Shin Nihon Chisso rōdō kumiai kikanshi, *Sairen*, no. 1931, August 31, 1968.

75. "The workers and fishers stand on the same ground as laborers. We support their struggle on principle. For practical support, the union, maintaining its independence, will do its best." *Shin Nitchitsu rōkumi nyūsu* (Shin Nitchitsu labor union news), August 20, 1959.

76. When scholars formed a research group in 1969 (first, *Saiban kenkyūkai,* or the Trial Research Group, later renamed as *Minamatabyō kenkyūkai,* or the Minamta Disease Research Group), Yamashita "worked in Chisso's Research Division" and "was one of several No. 1 union members who provided inside information from the company and participated in the [Research] group under assumed names." George, *Minamata*, 198–199.

77. "Zenkan-san ni haji sengen no koto o kiku" (Ask Zenkan-san about the Declaration of Shame). Yamashita Yoshihiro interviewed by Takakura Tsuzumiko and Takakura Souji, May 15, 2017, at Moyai Hall, Minamata. *Gaia Minamata,* June 30, 2017.

78. The union's earlier struggle against Chisso to realize a stable wage (*antei chingin*) may have paved a way for some union members to work with the fishers and sufferers in solidarity. This struggle resulted in a further division among the union members. When the union began to negotiate with the company for a stable wage in 1962, Chisso was in the midst of reducing the number of its employees, reflecting the declining sales of its products. For this purpose, the union was only an obstacle, and Chisso tried to diminish the union's influence over its employees. Then, the company created a second union to antagonize the original union while giving preferential treatment to the second union. For example, the company transferred the original union members to a place hard to commute to from home, relegated them to sections whose work did not reflect their special skills, and called for their early retirement. Some workers remembered the period as the most difficult time in Minamata's history because this wage stabilization struggle (*antei chingin tōsō or anchin tōsō*) divided employees and their family members; some stayed in the first union, while others left to the second. Members of the first union were marginalized at the Minamata factory. Those who were sidelined at work found their place in the Minamata Cultural Collective (*Minamata bunka shūdan*) and Citizens' Council for Minamata Disease Countermeasures (*Minamatabyō taisaku shimin kaigi*).

79. Weber, "Science as a Vocation," 133.

80. Jason Ā. Josephson-Storm, *The Myth of Disenchantment: Magic, Modernity, and the Birth of the Human Sciences* (Chicago: The University of Chicago Press, 2017), 4–8.

81. I learned, however, that some scholars work on this subject matter, such as Jeffrey J. Kripal. For example, Jeffrey J. Kripal, *Authors of the Impossible: The Paranormal and the Sacred* (Chicago: University of Chicago Press, 2010).

82. Jane Bennett, *The Enchantment of Modern Life: Attachments, Crossings, and Ethics* (Princeton: Princeton University Press, 2001), 131.

83. Bennett, *The Enchantment of Modern Life,* 4.

84. Bennett, *The Enchantment of Modern Life,* 163.

Chapter 3

The World of the Minamata Fishers

Forgiveness, Gift (nosari), *and the Sugimoto Family*

In his 2006 collection of essays *Yomi no inu* (*A Dog of Hades*), photographer and writer Fujiwara Shin'ya recalls a train ride that he had taken half a century earlier, in 1962, bound for Tokyo from Moji, a city not far from Minamata, on the southern island of Kyushu. Fujiwara was preparing to enter into college life in Tokyo. After sleeping overnight on the train and having the next day's lunch on board, Fujiwara noted that twenty hours had already passed. Then Mt. Fuji appeared through the window, an image solemn and touching. Fujiwara knew that from here, several more hours of the journey lay ahead of him before he would arrive in Tokyo, his final destination.[1]

Even in 2019, taking the newly opened and now fastest line of the *shinkansen* or bullet train (inaugurated on March 12, 2011, one day after the earthquake in eastern Japan), the trip from Tokyo to Minamata still takes about six hours. As we saw in chapter 2, the geographical distance separating the Chisso factory in Minamata from the corporate headquarters in Tokyo fostered and furthered a psychological distance that divided the people in Minamata, reproducing a hierarchical order predicated modern market values which in turn bred an unsympathetic attitude toward, and even discrimination against, Minamata sufferers.

Focusing on the Sugimoto family, this chapter examines ways in which the psychological distance in a small fishing community led to the discriminatory treatment of Minamata sufferer Sugimoto Eiko and her family. That is, how the Sugimotos came to terms with the loss of their loved ones' lives, their health, and faith in their fellow fishers; and how they restored their relationships with their natural surroundings. Ultimately, the Sugimoto family would forgive Chisso and, perhaps surprisingly, come to an understanding of the disease as a "gift." Understandably, the family's forgiveness of Chisso confused other sufferers and their supporters and was not enthusiastically endorsed by many other Hongan no kai members.

But some members did come to embrace the Sugimotos' determination, even as they continued to grapple with how to understand their conclusion. Like these more skeptical members of Hongan no kai, I, too, find it difficult to entirely support the notion of forgiveness in this context. But in this chapter, I propose that this surprising and indeed enigmatic forgiveness may be understood from the perspective of the alternative ontology of janaka shaba, or a world otherwise. In offering my account, I turn to Jane Bennett's notion of the "agency of assemblages," to reveal how the sufferers' vision of this world otherwise contributes to an environmental ethics.

The alternative ontology of Hongan no kai's world otherwise coincides with a conception of human agency not as individuals but as assemblages. This conception counters the view of the person as an independent and autonomous being, solely responsible for the consequences of her decisions. Bennett's notion of the agency of assemblages extends Gilles Deleuze and Félix Guattari's ontological framework of assemblages as "ad hoc groupings of diverse elements, of vibrant materials of all sorts. Assemblages are living, throbbing confederations that are able to function despite the persistent presence of energies that confront them from within."[2] The Sugimotos' act of forgiving the perpetrators whose acts led to widespread suffering, and perceiving the disease as a "gift," I will argue, are productively understood in terms of this ontology of assemblages—an alternative ontology with important implications for environmental ethics.

The agency as assemblages calls into question, and perhaps even nullifies, the familiar norms that distinguish self from other in the Western philosophical tradition, which presumes the autonomy of discrete individuals. The Western conception of persons, which has prevailed in academia, is what Bennett refers to as an "autonomous kind of agency to which Augustine and Kant (or an omnipotent God) aspired."[3] Emmanuel Levinas has offered sustained and far-reaching critiques of this ontology of personhood and its presupposition of an autonomously willing self that asserts its primacy over the other and envisions the world as centering on itself.[4] As Levinas and Bennett demonstrate, addressing issues stemming from a self-centered (and ultimately anthropocentric) worldview requires a reconception of on[illegible] and the imagining of agency constituted otherwise.

In order to bring such insights to bear on the matter of Minamata dis[illegible] I open my discussion with a historical overview of food-consumption p[illegible] tices in the Japanese archipelago. This account provides context for und[illegible] standing the ideological underpinnings of widespread discrimination again[illegible] fishers and hunters in Japan. Following this account, I trace the biography of Eiko and the Sugimoto family, focusing on their notions of "gift" and "forgiveness." I conclude the chapter by applying Bennett's concept of the agency of assemblages in an examination of these notions, better to understand how they might contribute to the discourse of environmental ethics.

FISHERS, HUNTERS, AND RICE-CENTERED IDEOLOGY

Minamata fisher, sufferer, and founding member of Hongan no kai, Ogata Masato, recalls that his mother urged him not to take over his family's fishing business, but instead to pursue a vocation as a carpenter or plasterer. Though a fisher's wife herself, Ogata's mother often referred to fishers as *jushi kwanjin*. In the local Minamata dialect, *jushi* denotes a fisher. *Kwanjin* or *kanjin* originally indicated a Buddhist mendicant who collected donations to build or maintain temples, but eventually became a synonym for a "beggar." The phrase that Ogata's mother used thus means "a fisher-beggar."[5] Use of this common but condescending phrase long predated Minamata disease, and thus speaks to the internalized discriminatory views toward fishers and their families. Tracing the social status of fishers and hunters in the course of Japanese history will thus illuminate the rhetoric and implicit strategies of exclusion of the fishing and hunting population, which reinforced the prevailing hegemonic social order at the time of the outbreak of methylmercury poisoning in Minamata.

Scholars in Japanese studies have observed that the fields of Japanese religion and history have paid little attention to the lives of non-farmers. Books, articles, and conferences focusing on maritime history and religious culture around the Japanese archipelago have only recently become available.[6] Among these studies, the late historian Amino Yoshihiko's research is notable for our purposes. Amino observes that the term *hyakushō*, widely used as a synonym for "commoners" within both scholarly and everyday discourse, is generally taken to indicate rice farmers or peasants bound to the land—not, in other words, fishers and hunters.

Amino's critical archival research, however, discloses the wide variety of work in which hyakushō have in fact historically been engaged; indeed, according to Amino, the people referred to under the category hyakushō have embodied the term's root meaning: a "household of hundreds"—hundreds of jobs, multitudinous forms of work and livelihood. The general use of hyakushō has thus narrowed in meaning, effectively contributing to the image of Japan as a rice-centered country. Amino takes the fact that the term now signifies farmers—to the exclusion of fishers and hunters—to have an ideological basis.[7]

As Amino argues, then, the neglect of fishers and hunters in favor of rice farmers in Japanese society is reproduced in Japanese studies—a matter that may not be attributed to a lack of documentation alone. In the course of Japanese history, rice has occupied a special place; rice farming has been intimately associated with emperor worship, serving as a foundation of Japan's Shinto-based theocracy and thereby upholding the social order of Japanese society—a social order that functionally excludes fishers and hunters.[8] In order to understand the ideological basis of the exclusionary attitudes and practices that will eventually characterize social relations in Minamata, it will be helpful briefly to examine scholarly treatment of a few key historical documents. As we will see, the history of attitudes toward food in Japan has been complex and sometimes ambiguous.

Historian Harada Nobuo, author of the pioneering monograph *Rekishi no naka no kome to niku* (*Rice and Meat in [Japanese] History*), observes that the third-century Chinese *Book of Wei* describes people living in the Japanese archipelago as refraining from eating meat during periods of mourning. On the basis of this account, Harada concludes that when not in mourning, people on the archipelago would engage in meat-eating, though the frequency and scope of this practice are uncertain.[9] Folklore scholar Shibusawa Keizō[10] offers further perspective in his examination of *Engishiki*, a book recording early Shinto court rituals from the seventh to ninth centuries.[11] The food offerings to Shinto deities included not only rice and sake—goods deriving from the farmer's labors—but also products from the sea—salt, seaweed, bonito, abalone, and salmon.[12] Based upon this textual evidence, Shibusawa argues that goods derived from the sea—fish among them—were held in high regard in Shinto rituals of the time.[13] These studies indicate that eating meat—or at least fish—was practiced during the early period of the formation of the Shinto theocracy.

But a change was occurring even as *Engishiki* was being compiled in 907 CE. Although *Engishiki* records the use of animal meat in Shinto rituals, Hans Martin Krämer claims that political changes already beginning in the seventh century, as Buddhism's influence was on the rise, contributed to the creation of a taboo against eating animal meat. "After the establishment of the first centralized state based on Chinese models in the 7th century A.D. [*sic*] were efforts made to diffuse agriculture among all those parts of the islands considered part of the emperor's realm."[14] Under the new regime, in which the spread of agriculture coincided with the scope of imperial power, Emperor Tenmu pronounced a ban on the consumption of animal meat in 675 CE.[15] The banned animals were referred to as *gochiku,* a term deriving from Buddhism. The category gochiku comprised five animals: cow, horse, dog, monkey, and chicken. In the following year, 676, Emperor Tenmu issued his first *Hōjōrei* (release order) for the release of fish and other captured animals—a ritual to atone for taking the lives of fish and other animals. Such occasional Hōjōrei indicates that taking the lives of animals is an action that, while necessary, also requires atonement.

Eventually, animal meat—wild boar, deer, and fish—was banned from Shinto ritual offerings. While Buddhism taught that eating meat was contrary to *ahimsa* (nonviolence toward living creatures), Shinto defined meat-eating as impure, and thus a defilement, associating it with blood and death.[16] Let alone the cadaver, coming into contact with blood, called *ketsue,* was a prominent social taboo. With the Buddhist proscription on taking lives and the Shinto prohibition of blood pollution in ritual contexts, the moral aversion to eating animals was transferred to avoidance of people responsible for hunting and capturing those animals. And as the above account further suggests, Temmu's authority extended to control of his subjects' dietary habits. The elevation of rice as a food of central importance emerges in this political context.

Anthropologist Peter Knecht summarizes this matter, noting that "it is no exaggeration to say that rice, since early in Japan's history, has been a symbol of power—religious power, yes, but even more political power—and a symbol of social distinction between those who wielded power from [*sic*] those who were 'guided' by that power."[17] As the emperor's power was consolidated and secured through promoting rice and presiding over its consecration rituals, meat-eating practices were denigrated, and those whose livelihoods involved capturing animals for food were consigned to a correspondingly lower social stratus.

Even as imperial reign was challenged and its political influence declined following the twelfth century, the sociomoral status to which fishers and hunters were relegated remained diminished. As Harada observes, *Shōjin gyorui monogatari* (*Tale of vegetarian fare and fishes*), a popular didactic folk tale from the fifteenth century, includes the story of a band of personified vegetables defeating a group of fish in battle.[18] Scholar of Buddhism Barbara Ambros has assembled a list of the constituents of each of the opposed "armies" in the folk tale: "The vegetarian army consists of soybean products, various vegetables, seaweed, and fruit, while the army of fish includes fish, shellfish, fowl, and game, but not large domestic animals, such as cattle or horses." The composition of these armies illustrates the line of demarcation separating categories of foods, and therefore their producers, in the popular imagination.[19] The conclusion to the tale, which sees the vegetable army winning over the animal army, indicates by extrapolation the relative social statuses of the food producers: vegetables and farmers are positioned as morally superior to animals, hunters, and fishers.

Japanese folklore scholar Nakamura Ikuo notes that such sociomoral hierarchies may also be observed in medieval Noh plays, such as *Utou*, *Ukai*, and *Akogi*, revealing popular perceptions of fishers and hunters during this period. All three stories depict punishments for taking the lives of animals. In *Utou*, a hunter descends to hell upon his death where utou birds attack him by the iron beaks and lead claws. In *Ukai*, a fisher is doomed to hell, saved only by the salvific power of the Lotus Sutra. *Akogi* provides a slightly more nuanced account, which includes a Shinto directive.[20] In this play, a fisher, upon his death, is punished in hell, not merely because his occupation entails killing fish, but also because he caught fish from a sanctuary, designated by Ise Shinto shrine, where fishing was forbidden. Despite the proscription on fishing, the fisher had continued to catch fish—not on behalf of others, but for his own consumption—a double transgression for which he is punished.[21] These popular stories all suggest that fishers (or hunters) deserve punishment; *Akogi* in particular describes the fisher as both sacrilegious and greedy.[22]

These examples convey the general perception of fishers (as well as hunters) in Japan; the low social status of fishers is justified through descriptions of their dubious moral character and underwritten by Buddhist and Shinto teachings. Such perceptions have proven to be long lived and pervasive, as indicated by the low esteem in which fishers were held in modern Minamata. The moral norms and related social order conveyed in the various texts discussed above inflected popular views of fishers, thereby contributing to discriminatory attitudes against them. But as we will soon see, fishers in Minamata have a religious culture of their own, a robust world that includes a sea god and other spirited entities.

Okamoto Tatsuaki, oral history collector, former Chisso employee, and chair of the First Labor Union (*daiichi kumiai*), whom we met in chapter 2, observes that discrimination against fishers tended to be more intense in areas where they were the new settlers. Okamoto notes that villagers called fishers *kara fuyuji*. *Fuyuji* refers to being lazy, and *kara* is an intensifier; kara fuyuji thus translates as "an extremely lazy person/people."[23] Ishimure Michiko recalls her painful encounter with medical doctors who expressed prejudice against Minamata fishers at the outbreak of Minamata disease and amid the fishers' riots (which we will examine in chapter 5). According to her account, not only did these doctors regard fishers as uneducated and unsophisticated; they also perceived the protesting fishers as a monolithic collective, not as humans—a mob with a temper, reacting not rationally, but purely on the basis of emotion.[24]

Sugimoto Takeshi, Eiko's husband, speaks to institutional discrimination against fishers: "The Japanese government has been discriminating against fishers. They would not listen to what [Minamata] fishers said, and this is how they have treated us. They do not regard fishers as humans."[25] Echoing Takeshi, Ogata Masato commented that rice farmers received financial support when the price of their products slumped in the market or when the government implemented a policy to control market prices, reducing rice-production acreage (*gentan seisaku*) to offset excessive harvests, whereas fishers never received any aid from the central government, regardless of the size of their catch.[26] Moreover, in light of the government's generous treatment of farmers, agricultural cooperatives throughout Japan have generally voted for the leading Liberal Democratic Party (LDP), and in turn, the LDP offers preferential treatment to farmers.

As we have seen, though some Buddhist and Shinto teachings suggest that fishers deserve punishment for carrying out their vocation, fishers have their own religious cosmologies, tropes, and rituals, deriving from Shinto, Buddhism, Daoism, and local folklore. Among fishers' various renditions of religious practices, perhaps the most notable and commonly observed is Ebisu worship.[27] Scholar of Japanese religions Fabio Rambelli identifies Ebisu as one of the popular sea gods, along with Watatsumi, Konpira, and the Chinese goddess Mazu (Maso or Seibo in Japanese).[28] One contemporary and prevalent image of Ebisu is found in the logo for the beer brand Yebisu, where the deity is depicted holding a sea bream and a fishing rod, conveying its closeness with fishing culture (Figure 3.1).

One of the origin stories of Ebisu is found in Shinto mythology. Ebisu was the first child born of Izanagi and Izanami, among the seventh generation of Shinto deities, believed to have given birth to many other deities as well as the islands of Japan. According to the myth, in the initial stages of courtship, Izanami, the female deity, spoke first to Izanagi, which was considered a breach of etiquette. As a result of this transgression, their first child was born

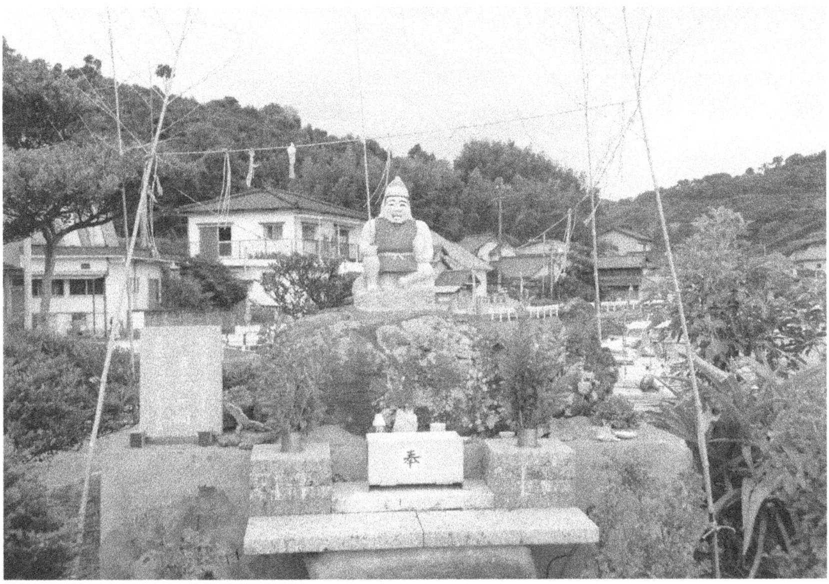

Figure 3.1 Ebisu Statue in Modō Area, Minamata. *Source:* Photo courtesy of Dr. Mark Hudson.

with missing limbs. Izanagi and Izanami abandoned this *hiruko* (leech child) by setting him afloat at sea.

In one variation of the mythic tale, Ebisu is believed to be this hiruko, who has drifted back to shore, bearing a large catch of fish. Rambelli explains the link between Ebisu and the drifting god at sea: "In many fishing communities, the god Ebisu was identified, more or less explicitly, with the fish they caught (whales, dolphins, salmon, etc.); in other communities, Ebisu was more generally associated with objects that would drift ashore from the sea—tree logs and various other items, even including corpses."[29] In his association with hiruko as a drifter at sea, Ebisu symbolizes the ambivalence of nature, as both a source of life, providing food to humans, and as a destroyer of life, engulfing humans, their boats, and houses along the shore. Ebisu thus embodies the "possibilities and ambivalence of the sea" as "a repository of untold riches and, at the same time, a disposal site for pollution and a very dangerous place."[30] Having been abandoned at sea due to its deformation, but returning with an abundant catch, Ebisu embodies dual aspects of nature. As illustrations of Ebisu holding a red snapper suggest, the deity could help bring the boons of nature in the form of a good catch, affirming fishers' livelihood.

Fishers in Minamata believe not only in the spirits inhering in natural phenomena like the sea but also in the spirits within human-made objects, for example, *funadama* (the spirit of the boat). Each boat has an altar for funadama, where people offer saké or food to the spirit.[31] As with Ebisu, fishers appeal to funadama for good catches and to protect the crew from storms and wrecks. Perceiving their boats as spirited rather than lifeless objects conveys an ontological view in which agency is not limited to humans but extends to nonhumans and other-than-humans. This religious perception, we will now see, is integral to Hongan no kai's worldview as well as the Sugimotos' attitude toward Minamata disease.

SUGIMOTO SUSUMU AND EIKO: MINAMATA DISEASE AS A *NOSARI* (GIFT)

Sugimoto Eiko (hereafter referred to by her given name, Eiko, so as to distinguish her from others in her family) was born in 1938, the only child of an *amimoto* family in Modō, Minamata. *Amimoto* literally means the source of a (fishing) net, signifying a chief of fishers who works together with the *amiko,* or children of a fishing net. In addition to providing a boat, nets, and fish spears, amimoto cares for fishers and their families as if they were his own family.[32] Eiko fondly recalls her life prior to Minamata disease in Modō, where four amimoto households worked together with around 120 amiko and their families.[33] As a leader of fishers, an amimoto is well respected among fishing families; Eiko's father, Susumu, who generally oversaw twenty to thirty amiko, was likewise respected.

As early as 1942, the fishers in Minamata and others in the vicinity took notice of the unprecedented symptoms of the disease that would come to be named after their town, first appearing among cats that bumped into people's legs, danced oddly, and drove themselves into the sea, drowning. Such phenomena intensified in the early 1950s, when humans began to show similar symptoms—losing control over their bodies, falling, tipping over, and shaking violently, thereby rendering them incapable of speaking or swallowing food. Beginning in 1954, residents of Modō also began to notice bizarre behavior among local cats. By 1958, Eiko's mother, Toshi, who had been always healthy, cheerful, and energetic enough to take care of many amiko, began to complain of pains in her body.[34]

One day, having returned from fishing, Eiko found Toshi sitting in the middle of the front yard, surrounded by a number of burned matches scattered on the ground. When Eiko approached her from behind and turned Toshi's head, she found Toshi's face covered with blisters. When asked what had happened, Toshi replied that she had merely tried to light a *kiseru* (a smoke pipe) with a match but had lost control of her hands. Instead of lighting the kiseru, she kept pushing the lit matches into her face. After this incident, Eiko's father Susumu took Toshi to Minamata City Hospital, where she was immediately sent to the isolation ward. Not knowing the cause of her symptoms, but having seen many other patients exhibiting similar behaviors, the doctors suspected that Toshi had contracted a *kibyō* (strange disease) that they believed might be contagious. According to Ishimure Michiko, the isolation ward had a history of abandoning patients with contagious illnesses or mental disturbances, receiving no visits from doctors.[35] The sick patients were confined to rooms where they lay on wooden floors, awaiting only their deaths.

It was at this hospital that Eiko saw other sufferers in grave condition. Some were constrained on their beds, so as not to hurt themselves with their uncontrollable gestures, while others, overpowered by a hyperbolic energy, incessantly ran at full speed from one corner to another before hitting the walls hard enough to knock themselves unconscious. Seizures, a common symptom, made it difficult for patients to keep down their food. Consequently, in some cases, a combination of physical exhaustion and malnutrition led to death, the patients' bodies diminished to skin and bones.[36]

Upon Toshi's hospitalization, the local radio announced that she suffered from manganese poisoning—the initial, and mistaken, diagnosis for the "strange disease." Once Toshi's illness was made public, the Sugimotos' lives were upended, and their whole community transformed. Lacking adequate and accurate knowledge of the illness, people feared it was contagious. Consequently, others in the community avoided contact with the Sugimoto family, shunning all its members, even verbally and physically harassing them. The residents justified their acts of ostracism and harassment with claims that Toshi's disease had harmed the sales of their catch at the market.

"I cried listening to the radio news [of Toshi's diagnosis], for manganese poisoning was considered to be incurable at the time," recalled Eiko, "and not a single person visited our house to console us after the broadcast, which was also painful. People who had had supper with us on the previous night never again set foot into our house. Back then, the belief that the disease was contagious changed the community members' attitude toward us completely."[37] Susumu would visit Toshi at the hospital every day, bringing Eiko. When many people still thought of the illness as transmissible, Susumu often said, "I don't mind catching her disease."[38] But Eiko recalled that one day, she and her father went out to visit their relatives. When they were approaching the house, a relative yelled at them, "Shame on you! Never come near us!"[39]

Curiously, the eventual discovery of the actual cause of the disease—methylmercury poisoning from Chisso's wastewater—did not change people's treatment of the Sugimotos. To visit Toshi in the hospital, Eiko and Susumu had to take a path concealed behind bushes, rather than walking on a paved street, for fear that exposure might invite verbal and physical attacks from other residents. Deprived of his identity as an amimoto, Susumu told Eiko that if the three of them—Susumu, Toshi, and Eiko—died together of the same disease, he would have nothing to regret, however excruciating the illness might be.[40] In the same year as Toshi's hospitalization in 1959, Eiko married Takeshi, who was not a fisher, and adopted his family name. By this time, Eiko was also exhibiting symptoms, becoming weak and frequently stumbling.

After three miscarriages, Eiko gave birth to her first son with Takeshi in 1961. To the Sugimoto family's happiness, she had four further sons who showed no trace of methylmercury poisoning. With each labor and birth, oddly enough, Eiko felt healthier and healthier. For a long time, the medical community had subscribed to the hypothesis that mercury (or any chemicals) would not travel through an umbilical cord; thus, a fetus in the mother's womb would be unaffected by poisons. The theory was used to deny any attribution of a newborn baby's ill health to methylmercury poisoning. However, a devoted doctor in Kumamoto, Harada Masazumi, discovered that methylmercury could indeed be transferred from a mother's body to her fetus. Since methylmercury moved through her body, each pregnancy reduced the amount of accumulated methylmercury in Eiko's body. Harada had discovered the explanation for Eiko's restored health.

Upon the birth of Eiko's first son, the hospital gave Toshi permission to go home for a few days to see her grandson. On the evening of her return home, Toshi went out for a walk for the first time in many months. Not long after she embarked on her walk, Eiko and Takeshi, who were waiting for her at home, heard Toshi scream from the direction of the beach. They dashed out to find Toshi alone at the edge of a cliff. According to Toshi, a man had approached her from behind and pushed her, nearly causing her to fall into the sea. Fortunately, she was able to cling to the ground and was rescued, uninjured. The man who had attacked her was not a stranger but an acquaintance, for whom Toshi served as a go-between.[41] When Eiko and Takeshi confronted the attacker, he replied, "You shouldn't walk around in our community. When *you* are out being seen, it is *us* who suffer the consequences."[42] Soon after this incident, Toshi passed away. But the violence did not cease. Eiko's longtime friend Ishimure Michiko recalls visiting Eiko at her house, where windows had been broken by anonymous attackers, leaving shards on the tatami mat.[43]

The situation grew worse when Susumu decided to file a lawsuit against Chisso in 1969. His patience with ten years of negligence by Chisso and the abusive treatment by his fellow villagers had worn out. "Never have I harmed nor bullied others in my life," said Susumu in an uncharacteristically strong tone, "yet we are thrown into an unbearable condition. I cannot die until I make clear whose fault this is to the public eye."[44] The initial lawsuit was called *daiichiji soshō* (the first trial); it was followed by several others. Susumu became the first plaintiff in the Modō community to file a lawsuit, similar to a class-action, against Chisso.[45]

Believing that the lawsuit would further decrease the market price of their catches, fishers in the community threatened the Sugimotos: "Don't count on the moon shining on you at night. Be alert at night with no moon."[46] Once tightly knit and forming a quasi-family, the community was broken up by the disease and further shattered by the lawsuit. Some former fishers found new means of making a living, leaving the community for good, while others went to work for Chisso. Eiko recalled that Chisso lured many amiko to its side: "We will hire you since you cannot fish. No examination will be given to work for us."[47] With no need to invest in a boat or a fishing net, no fear of the market price ever declining, and no training required for employment, Chisso's offer was quite attractive to amiko fishers in the community who were struggling to make ends meet since the advent of the strange disease. Exploiting the rift in the community, Chisso effectively ensured that members of this precarious population would antagonize one another instead of fighting in solidarity against Chisso and the government.[48]

Chisso did not leave the Sugimotos alone, either. A man in a business suit, which in Minamata could only signify a Chisso employee, would visit the Sugimotos and try to cajole them to withdraw from the lawsuit, bribing them with cash. Eiko's family never gave in to these aggressive advances. At one point, Chisso convinced Eiko's relatives to attempt to persuade her family to withdraw the lawsuit, with threats of violence if necessary. In a conversation with Eiko, Ishimure learned of one of Eiko's most troubling memories: "Once, my uncle came to our house. He had a broad-bladed kitchen knife in his hand, pointing it at me."[49] He had been sent by Chisso to terrorize Eiko into abandoning the lawsuit. On another occasion, Chisso had the villagers cut up the Sugimotos' fishing nets. Nets were not only valuable resources for the fishers; fishers were also often emotionally attached to the tools of their trade. On yet a different occasion, the Sugimotos' fishing boat was stolen and taken for a joyride. Riding in someone's boat without permission was a public insult and humiliation. It took a few days to repair the broken nets, but it took far more time for the Sugimotos to recover from the emotional wound and the blow to their pride as fishers.[50] On hearing Eiko's testimony, Ishimure struck a somber note that undercuts any romantic notion of a harmonious fishing village: "A community is not always rosy."[51]

Under such circumstances, Eiko believed that although Minamata disease was indeed a fearful thing, people were more frightening than the illness. In an ironic twist, those who wronged the Sugimotos would themselves succumb to the disease, dying excruciating deaths one by one. Even when, for his and his family's safety, he had to confine himself to his house, with all its doors and windows locked, Susumu never spoke ill of others, telling Eiko the people in the community were upright and righteous, despite their maltreatment of his family. Notwithstanding his physical torment from Minamata disease and his emotional distress from the community's abuse, Susumu continued to insist that no one should try to change others, nor take revenge upon those who have perpetrated agonies; rather, one should focus on changing oneself. To Eiko's disbelief—though eventually she would embrace Susumu's sentiments—Susumu even described Toshi's illness as a *nosari* (gift). Knowing his nature, it should have come as no surprise, Eiko later thought,[52] but this was beyond her comprehension at the time.

Gift and the Agency of Assemblages

Nosari is a word rich in meaning. Eiko remembered various occasions when her father used the term. For example, Susumu never described a large catch as *tairyō*, a word commonly used for an ample haul. Instead, he and other Minamata fishers used the word nosari. When Susumu caught a substantial amount of fish, he would say, "*Okagesama de nosatta zo*" ("I am grateful for the nosari"), employing a verb form of nosari. Similarly, the fishers would not say *furyō* (a poor catch); instead, they would comment that they did not deserve nosari that day. Nosari is also used to refer to things and situations beyond gifts from the sea. On his deathbed, Susumu told Eiko, "Think of it as a nosari if you get a disease like your mother,"[53] indicating that Toshi's illness was a nosari, and so was his own.

Eiko eventually realized that Susumu meant that despite the Sugimotos becoming victims of Minamata disease, to be a victim is better than to be a victimizer.[54] To Susumu's mind, not being a victimizer had nothing to do with the virtue of one's character. Rather, it was a matter of sheer nosari. If some other amiko family had fallen ill first, Susumu, out of fear of catching the same disease, might have behaved like others around him, shunning and bullying the sufferers and the entire family. Minamata disease prompted Susumu to reevaluate his role as an amimoto. Taking pride in being an amimoto, Susumu would tell Eiko that "amimoto must love people," even those who have done wrong.[55] Indeed, he perceived Minamata disease as a spiritual trial: How can one love those who ostracized and violently attacked one and one's property?

In order to address this question, we should investigate why and how the idea of perceiving a disease, harassment, and violence as nosari emerged. Such study may help us understand the religious sensibility that enables Susumu, Eiko, and other Minamata fishers to relate to nonhumans and other-than-humans, which will in turn serve as the foundation of a world otherwise in which no one is either victim or victimizer.

To this end, discussing a few further aspects of the Sugimotos' relationship to the sea will be helpful. Although bioaccumulation of methylmercury in the waters around them had made them ill, Minamata fishers never lost their intimacy with the sea and their natural surroundings. Eiko fondly recalls that her father often told her that although they had *gyogyōken* (the legal right to catch fish in a designated area), the sea did not belong to the fishers but to the fish and all the other beings in the sea.[56] Eschewing anthropocentrism, their worldview centered on creatures of the sea. A natural consequence of this attitude is that Eiko referred to fish by using the honorary but simultaneously intimate suffix *–don*, derived from *tono* (the lord), as a token of respect for the fish. Referring to fish (*uo*) as "*uo-don*," speaks to a perspective in which humans are not sovereign over the world of the sea, and the sea's creatures are not their property. Humans do not constitute the center of this world(view); in fact, the world thus envisioned had no "center," but encompasses multitudinous beings consisting of nonhumans and perhaps even other-than-humans, such as Ebisu. Their heterogeneous, enspirited world is characterized not by a "strong, autonomous kind of agency,"[57] but by the agency of assemblages.[58]

Seeing himself as part of an assemblage of beings, Susumu developed rituals to express his gratitude to the sea. He would offer saké to the sea in the beginning of the seaweed season, asking for a good harvest. Again, at the end of the season, he would offer saké to the sea and the fish, thanking them for nourishing him, his family, and the community.[59] For him, this was a way of communicating with nonhumans and other-than-humans, maintaining intimacy with the world of which he was a part.

Fishers' relations are not limited to the water but extend to rivers, mountains, and all their natural surroundings—a key aspect of the agency of assemblages. As Eiko recounts, her grandparents and her parents—all fishers—told her repeatedly to take good care of the trees in the mountains.[60] This concern for care of the natural environment arises from a worldview in which trees, mountains, and the sea are perceived as interconnected assemblages. Eiko's fellow Minamata fisher Ogata Masato explains:

> Planting a tree in the mountains controls the flow of water. The rain falls in the mountains, and a river runs through the mountains, flowing into the Shiranui Sea. Trees shepherd the rain into the soil. Once the trees are gone, the rainwater will not be retained but will run through the soil's surface, eroding it. As a result, the muddy water would lead to the seaweeds' disappearance, and the absence of minerals in the water deposited in a deeper layer of the mountain soil would bring a noticeable change in the sea's ecosystem when it flows into the sea.[61]

In contrast to the water that seeps into the soil, enriching it with minerals, muddy water running from the surface of the mountain into the sea suffocates seaweed. When the trees cover the mountains, their roots retain the rainwater in the ground, which eventually flows into the river and the sea. By the time the water reaches the Shiranui Sea, it carries abundant nutritious minerals from the soil. The minerals enrich the water, nourish the seaweed, and foster the sea's biodiversity.[62] The sea, thus enriched, nurtures a wild variety of fish.

Ogata's observations about the gift from the sea make clear that such a gift is not unilateral but rather a collaboration among multiple entities: the rainfall, the mountains, the minerals in the soil, the river that carries them, and so on. The Sugimotos and Ogata live in such a world in which agencies are imagined not atomistically, but "as distributive and confederate."[63] According to Jane Bennett, such agencies are "distributed across a mosaic, but it is also possible to say something about the kind of striving that may be exercised by a human within the assemblage."[64] This striving, we will see in the chapters that follow, constitutes a key element of the ontology of a world otherwise.

Earlier I expressed my hesitation to embrace the view on Minamata disease as a nosari, since the idea may lead to failures to identify the cause of the harm and failure to impute to the victimizers' responsibility necessary for adjudicating restitution. Acknowledging the possible pitfalls of this imagination of the collective agency of assemblages, Bennett writes:

> such a notion broadens the range of places to look for sources [of harmful effects]. Look to long-term strings of events: to selfish intentions, to energy policy offering lucrative opportunities for energy trading while generating a tragedy of the commons, and to a psychic resistance to acknowledging a link between American energy use, American imperialism, and anti-Americanism;

> but look also to the stubborn directionality of a high-consumption social infrastructure, to unstable electron flows, to conative wildfires, to exurban housing pressures, and to the assemblages they form.[65]

Bennett thus defends the idea of the agency of assemblages on the grounds that it would in fact help reveal structural problems, enabling one to address fundamental issues—not merely symptoms—and thereby help avoid the recurrence of tragedy. In other words, embracing the agency of assemblages does not preclude imputation of responsibility for irrevocable damage. On the contrary, whereas the "modern" system has failed to impute responsibility for such harm, approaching ethical matters through the framework of the agency of assemblages helps reveal the "crosscurrents" that give rise to catastrophe.

Whatever reservations one may have concerning Susumu's worldview, including his conception of Minamata disease as a nosari, it should urge us to seek a new ontological vision, one that would correct and protect against the damages wrought by our modern, anthropocentric ontology. Regarding Minamata disease as a nosari without an understanding of this call for a new ontology is treacherous, for it results in preventing the perpetrators from facing their own actions, while failing to redress culpability at a structural level. But what the Sugimotos' plight and their resilience offers is a model for an ontological shift toward the vision of a world otherwise. In chapter 4, I will further engage the discussion of the agency of assemblages as a new ethical element, bringing fisher and Minamata sufferer Ogata Masato's thoughts into dialogue with the work of philosopher Giorgio Agamben.

NOTES

1. Fujiwara, Shin'ya, *Yomi no inu* (*A Dog of Hades*) (Tokyo: Bungei shunjū, 2006), 16–17. Fujiwara suggested that the blindness of Matsumoto Chizuo, the leader of Aum Shinrikyō (which perpetrated the sarin gas attack in the Tokyo subway in 1995), might have been caused by mercury poisoning from Chisso.
2. Bennett, *Vibrant Matter*, 23–24.
3. Bennett, *Vibrant Matter*, 36.
4. Emmanuel Levinas criticized Western philosophy as "egology," as such, a philosophy of "power," and advocates a new kind of ontology, in which the self and the other have an asymmetrical relation. Levinas, *Totality and Infinity*, 46, 48.
5. Kaneko Akira and Oda Junko, interview by Ogata Masato and Kanazashi Junpei, "Koshikoba ni kite 17nen: sukoshi wa kioi ga toretakana" ("Seventeen Years Have Passed Since We Moved to Koshikoba: We Are Now Less Worked Up") *Tamashii utsure* 44 (2011): 16.
6. In the field of anthropology, Yanagita Kunio studied the fishers' lives in the early twentieth century and was followed by several scholars, including Miyamoto Tsuneo. A recent article by Yasumuro Satoru is also quite informative regarding

the lives of fishers and further obscures the divisions between fishers and farmers. Yasumuro Satoru, "'Hyakushō ryōshi' to 'Ryōshi hyakushō': Umitsuki no mura no seigyō fukugou to suiden inasaku" ("Farming Fisherman and Fishing Farmer: Subsistence Composition and a Paddy Field in the Sea Village") *Kokuritsu rekishi minzoku hakubutsukan kenkyū hōkoku* 162 (2011): 323–343. In the field of history, Kojima, Takeshi edited a book series, *Higashi ajia kaiiki ni kogidasu* (*Rowing the East Asian Ocean*) (Tokyo: Tokyo daigaku shuppankai, 2013), and Fabio Rambelli compiled various scholars' essays in *The Sea and the Sacred in Japan: Aspects of Maritime Religion* (London: Bloomsbury, 2018).

7. Amino, Yoshihiko, *Kaimin to Nihonshakai* (*The Maritime People and Japanese Society*) (Tokyo: Shin jinbutsu oraisha, 2009 [1998]), 47. His argument would also unsettle the geopolitical boundaries along modern nation-state lines that have confined academic studies

8. On this point, see also Harada, Nobuo, *Rekishi no naka no kome to niku: Shokumotsu to ten'no/sabetsu* (*Rice and Meat in History: Food, Emperor, and Discrimination*) (Tokyo: Heibonsha, 2013 [2005]).

9. Harada, *Rekishi no naka no kome to niku*, 113–114.

10. He was also a banker and grandson of a leading business person in the Meiji era, Shibusawa Eiichi.

11. It was compiled in 927, followed by several revisions.

12. Shibusawa, Keizō, "Engishiki nai suisan shinsen ni kansuru kousatsu jakkan" ("A Study of Shinto Offerings of Marine Products in *Engishiki*") in *Shibusawa Keizō chosakushū* (The Collected works of Shibusawa Keizō), vol. 1 (Tokyo: Heibonsha, 1993), 491–536. Moreover, in Japan, salt was commonly made of sea water, since rock salt was rare.

13. To this day, we see the influence of this regard in the symbol of a type of gift wrapping, called *noshi,* that is derived from dried abalones (*noshi*), and *noshi bukuro,* meaning literally a pouch of *noshi,* is still used to envelop cash as a gift on such occasions as weddings, funerals, and the New Year. For example, see Harumi Befu, "Gift-Giving in A Modernizing Japan," *Monumenta Nopponica* 23, no. 4 (1968): 445–456.

14. Hans Martin Krämer, "'Not Befitting Our Divine Country': Eating Meat in Japanese Discourses of Self and Other from the Seventeenth Century to the Present," *Food and Foodways*, 16 (2008): 36.

15. The ban is mentioned in the chronicle *Nihon shoki* (compiled in 720). See Krämer, "'Not Befitting Our Divine Country,'" 36.

16. Harada, *Rekishi no naka no kome to niku*, 114–115.

17. Peter Knecht, "Rice Representations and Reality," *Asian Folklore Studies: Narratives and Rituals in Asian Folk Religion and Culture* 66 (2007): 22.

18. Harada, *Rekishi no naka no kome to niku*, 131.

19. Barbara R. Ambros, "Partaking of Life: Buddhism, Meat-Eating, and Sacrificial Discourses of Gratitude in Contemporary Japan," *Religions* 10, no. 4 (2019): 279, https://doi.org/10.3390/rel10040279. Ambros also noted that "fish, fowl, and game remained common food items" during this period.

20. Originally the name of an inlet, *Akogi ga ura,* but because of this story, *akogi* has come to mean greedy or importunate in the contemporary usage of the word.

21. Nakamura, Ikuo, *Saishi to Kugi: Nihonjin no shizenkan dōbutsukan* (*Ritual and Sacrifice: Japanese Views of Nature and Animals*) (Kyoto: Hōzōkan, 2001), 208–209.

22. A Jesuit missionary, Luís Fróis, who landed on the Japanese archipelago in 1563 and documented the people's lives in his numerous letters home, reported that he had been puzzled that while fishers were respected in Europe, their Japanese counterparts were considered base. Since *Akogi* had been played by the fifteenth century, the discriminatory attitude toward fishers was widely shared. Harada, *Rekishi no naka no kome to niku*, 236.

23. Okamoto, *Minamatabyō no minshūshi*, 40–41. *Kara* refers to ancient China, and the term is based on the derogatory term for the Chinese people.

24. Ishimure, Michiko, "Teidan 'Nochi no yo no inochi' ni mukete, Minamata to gendai" ("Roundtable, Toward 'Lives Yet to Come,' Minamata and the Present") *Tamashii utsure* 34 (2008): 18.

25. Sugimoto, Takeshi, "Hongan no kai zadankai: Tsukamidokoro no nai bakemono" ("Hongan no kai Roundtable: Unfathomable Monsters") *Tamashii utsure* 41 (2010): 21.

26. Sawahata, Tōru (Airinkan director), interviewed by Ogata Masato, "Ekorojī ni motozuku 'mura okoshi' to torikunde 16nen" ("Promoting an Ecological Development of the Area for the Past 16 Years") *Tamashii utsure* 43 (2010): 13.

27. Fabio Rambelli, "General Introduction: The Sea in the History of Japanese Religions," in *The Sea and the Sacred in Japan*, ed. Fabio Rambelli (London: Bloomsbury, 2018), xviii.

28. Rambelli, "General Introduction," xviii. However, Ebisu is also worshipped in places other than fishing communities, according to the musicologist Ōuchi Fumi, who listed some characteristic assigned to Ebisu: the "god of a good catch in fishing communities, the god of the rice fields in the countryside, and the protector of markets and merchants." Ōuchi Fumi, "Musical Instruments for the Sea-God Ebisu: The Mythological System of Miho Shrine and Its Performative Power," in *The Sea and the Sacred in Japan*, ed. Fabio Rambelli (London: Bloomsbury, 2018), 53.

29. Fabio Rambelli, "Sea Theologies: Elements for a Conceptualization of Maritime Religiosity in Japan," in *The Sea and the Sacred in Japan*, ed. Fabio Rambelli (London: Bloomsbury, 2018), 191.

30. Rambelli, "Sea Theologies," 191. The ambivalence of nature, specifically the sea, is observed in other parts of the world. Citing a newspaper article on people in the Kanyakumari district of the state of Tamil Nadu, India (the area devastated by the 2004 tsunami), the anthropologist Frédérique Apffel-Marglin stated, "For these traditional Indian fisherfolk, the sea is not a natural resource but rather is a goddess with whom they interact, whom they respect, whose gifts make them live, and to whom they reciprocate with gift offerings. The sacralization of the sea in no way means that it is not to be used. In fact, one could suggest the opposite: it is the bounty of the sea and its life-sustaining quality, as well as its destructive power, that are the central aspects of its sacrality. Apffel-Marglin, *Subversive Spiritualities*, 24.

31. Nelly Naumann, "Whale and Fish Cult in Japan: A Basic Feature of Ebisu Worship," *Asian Folklore Studies* 33, no. 1 (1974): 6–7.

32. Some amimoto own boats and provide nets but do not fish themselves, but Minamata amimoto are usually fishers themselves.

33. Sugimoto, Eiko, "Minamata byō to tomoni" ("Life with Minamata Disease") in *Shōgen Minamatabyō* (*Testimonies: Minamata Disease*), ed. Kurihara Akira (Tokyo: Iwanami shoten, 2011 [2000]), 130–131.

34. Sugimoto, "Minamata byō to tomoni," 132.

35. Ishimure Michiko, "Ten no taue" ("Rice Planting in Heaven") in *Tamashii no hikyō kara* (*From a Hidden Spot of the Spirit World*) (Tokyo: Asahi shimbunsha, 2018), 186.

36. Sugimoto, "Minamata byō to tomoni," 134

37. Sugimoto, "Minamata byō to tomoni," 133.

38. Yanagita Kunio, "Minamata kara no keiji, vol. 1, Modō, Umi no kotozute" ("The Revelation from Minamata, vol. 1, Modō, the Prophet from the Sea") *Tamashii utsure* 33 (2008): 25.

39. Sugimoto, "Minamata byō to tomoni," 133.

40. Sugimoto, "Minamata byō to tomoni," 133.

41. In arranged marriages, a couple is usually introduced by a go-between.

42. Sugimoto, "Minamata byō to tomoni," 135–136.

43. Ishimure, Michiko, "Minamata Mandara wakai hōkoku 'mirai e no teigen' katariau" ("Report from Minamata Mandala Talk Session Discussing 'Suggestions from the future'") *Tamashii utsure* 29 (2007): 17.

44. Sugimoto, "Minamata byō to tomoni," 136.

45. Strictly speaking, it differs from a class action in the United States where one can join anonymously the class-action lawsuit. The Japanese court does not approve anonymous plaintiffs.

46. Ishimure, "Minamata Mandara wakai houkoku," 27.

47. Sugimoto Eiko and Sugimoto Takeshi, "Sugimoto Eiko-san, Takeshi-san Kuamoto Gakuen dai Minamatagaku kouza de kataru" ("Sugimoto Eiko and Takeshi Talked in a Minamata Study Course Session at Kumamoto Gakuen University") *Tamashii utsure* 33 (2008): 15.

48. "Sugimoto Eiko-san, Takeshi-san," 16. This tactic of dividing the population against itself was also observable in Fukushima and elsewhere.

49. Ishimure Michiko, "Tamashii ga ozoburuu" ("The Spirit Is Trembling") *Tamashii utsure* 2 (2000): 15–16; Ishimure, "Minamata Mandara wakai hōkoku," 27.

50. Sugimoto, "Minamata byō to tomoni," 138.

51. Ishimure, "Minamata Mandara wakai hōkoku," 27.

52. "Sugimoto Eiko-san, Takeshi-san," 15–16.

53. Sugimoto, Eiko, "*Hongan no kai* zadankai 'inochi no negai' o motomete Minamata kara kangaeru" ("*Hongan no kai* Roundtable: Seeking a 'Vow for Life' from Minamata") *Tamashii utsure* 35 (2007): 17.

54. Sugimoto, "Minamata byō to tomoni," 141.

55. Sugimoto, "Minamata byō to tomoni," 141.

56. Sugimoto, Eiko, "Arigatou gisei no umini" ("Thank You for the Sacrificed Sea, Sugimoto Takeshi and Eiko interview by Kanazashi Junpei") *Tamashii utsure* 10 (2002): 6.

57. Bennett, *Vibrant Matter*, 36.

58. One of the masterpieces by the documentarian Tsuchimoto Noriaki, *Minamata*, vividly captures the fishers' relations to the sea and the fish. In one scene, an octopus catcher in a kitchen in his house cuts a fresh octopus that he has just caught in the bay. His hands quiver, suggesting that he is affected with mercury poisoning. Even knowing that the octopuses caught in Shiranui Sea contain some amounts of mercury, he says that he cannot stop catching them, since not catching them is not communicating with them. Leaving his occupation would mean abandoning the octopus and other beings in the sea, and severing the relationship with them would be the loss of himself, as he can be himself only in interaction with others—the octopus and sea. Tsuchimoto's camera follows him standing in the water waist deep when catching octopus. It is striking to see his unadulterated smile at the camera, while holding an octopus in his hand. For this octopus catcher, the sea and the nonhumans in the sea are more than what he owes his life and livelihood but of which he is a part. It is important to emphasize that although moved by this octopus catcher, by no means do I endorse the consumption of unsafe food, as was rekindled after the Fukushima accident. Tsuchimoto Noriaki, *Minamata: The Victims and Their World*, 1971. Timothy Morton explains such sensitivity as follows: "We realize that nonhuman entities exist that are incomparably more vast and powerful than we are, and that our reality is caught in them. . . . For the modernist mind, accustomed to systems and structures, this is an astounding, shocking discovery. The more map we make, the more real things tear through them. Nonhuman entities emerge through our mapping, then they destroy them. Coexistence is in our face: it *is* our face. We are made of nonhuman and nonsentient and nonliving entities. It's not a cozy situation: it's a spooky, uncanny situation." Morton, *Hyperobjects*, 130.

59. Sugimoto, Eiko, "Arigatou gisei no umini" 6.

60. Sugimoto, Eiko, "Umetaterareta haha naru umi" ("Mother Sea Landfilled") *Tamashii utsure* 3 (2000): 9.

61. Sawahata, "Ekorojī ni motozuku," 8.

62. Hatakeyama Shigeatsu is an oyster and scallop farmer in Kesen'numa in the northern part of Japan, but his idea, shared by many fishers throughout Japan, was published and became known. To recover an environment that would nurture and maintain the rich biodiversity in the sea, he began to plant trees. Hatakeyama's writings include *Mori wa umi no koibito* (*The woods Are the Sea's Lover*) (Tokyo: Bungei shunjū, 2006) and *Mori wa tetsu de yomigaeru* (*Iron Will Resuscitate the Woods*) (Tokyo: Bungei shunjū, 2012).

63. Bennett, *Vibrant Matter*, 38.

64. Bennett, *Vibrant Matter*, 38.

65. Bennett, *Vibrant Matter*, 37.

Chapter 4

Before Good and Evil

*Ogata Masato on Spirit/*Tamashii

On March 17, 2017, the Maebashi district civil affairs court in Gunma prefecture handed down a guilty verdict, finding TEPCO and the Japanese government accountable for the Fukushima Daiichi nuclear power plant meltdown in 2011, disclosing that the defendants had foreseen the possibility of a catastrophic tsunami hitting the plant as early as 2002.[1] The case, filed by 137 Fukushima evacuees, demanded 1.5 billion Japanese yen as compensation for their relocation and emotional distress. Despite the plaintiffs' victory, disappointment and concerns remained. The judgment set the compensation much lower than the sum the plaintiffs had sought. At the same time, TEPCO appealed to a higher court, wishing to avoid admission of wrongdoing and claiming the compensation was too high. Meanwhile, uneven distribution of the compensation monies, doled out according to proximity to the plant, threatened to divide the plaintiffs against each other. Finally, as noted in a newspaper article following the trial, "Only a few of [the plaintiffs] have made their names public out of concern for possible discrimination against their children and negative effects on their jobs. . . . [One of the plaintiffs reports accusatory words from her neighbor] 'You can get money if you go to court, can't you?'"[2] In other words, the plaintiffs were regarded with suspicion, as if they had exaggerated their hardships out of pecuniary avarice.

This court decision was the first of thirty such "class-action suits filed nationwide involving more than 10,000 plaintiffs."[3] Among these lawsuits, a case filed by *Fukushima genpatsu kokusodan*, or Complainants for Criminal Prosecution of the Fukushima Nuclear Disaster (hereafter "Complainants"), headed by Mutō Ruiko, was remarkable for being able to file not a civil affair but a criminal lawsuit. This lawsuit sought not only compensation, but attempted to establish the "truth about responsibility" for "the prevention of a future repetition." To this end, the Complainants' priority was to see the accused acknowledge their accountability and to ensure "mitigation of ongoing harm."[4]

In her article "From Fukushima," Norma Field details the vicissitudes of the Complainants' path to bringing this charge to court. The Complainants had to remove the names of thirty individuals from their criminal charges in order to narrow the focus of the case, thereby helping ensure the case would be taken up by the court. This action left only three individuals as defendants. After these practical yet painful decisions, the Complainants learned that the local Fukushima prosecutors had declined to hear the Complainants' case, claiming that they found no evidence of criminality; the prosecutors deemed the meltdown to have been caused by an unpreventable force, not by the defendants' negligence around safety measures. The Complainants then turned to the *Kensatsu shinsakai,* the Committee for the Inquest of Prosecution, to determine whether the prosecutors' decision was appropriate. This action was brought to the Tokyo District public prosecutors, only to be dismissed. Finally, a new Committee for the Inquest of Prosecution agreed to undertake the case, and it was with this turn that the lawsuit began. It was thus five years after the meltdown that the case was finally brought to the court. It would be another three years before the final verdict was issued in 2019. To the great disappointment of the Complainants and their supporters, the court acquitted the TEPCO executives.[5]

Facing a charge of "professional negligence resulting in the deaths of 44 people who were forced to evacuate from a hospital near the plant and injuries to others,"[6] Katsumata Tsunehira, one of the three TEPCO executives on trial, issued an apology. While expressing his regret, he nonetheless rebuffed the charge leveled at him: "I would like to offer fresh apologies for the serious accident and the extensive trouble experienced by people surrounding the plant and the broader public. . . . But I believe that it was impossible to foresee such a tsunami and accident back then."[7]

Indeed, the most contested matter in this trial concerned the predictability of a large-scale tsunami in connection with the risks posed by the operation of a nuclear power plant that might be structurally vulnerable to such a force. In a "risk society"—Ulrich Beck's term for the unavoidable risks of modernization[8]—Katsumata's statement gives rise to questions pertinent to Minamata as well: What does it mean for one to apologize even as one refuses to recognize fault for one's decisions and behaviors? What does it mean to be held responsible for an event that is inevitable yet irrevocable in a risk society that includes such things as nuclear power plants' accidents? And what should we expect legal procedures to produce in cases of destruction of life and livelihood?

Bearing in mind the ongoing issues in Fukushima, this chapter addresses complex questions about responsibility in regard to Minamata disease. As we noted in chapter 3, the agency of assemblages that characterizes the ontological shift of *janaka shaba*, or a world otherwise, raises the question of moral responsibility. While the agency of assemblages may obscure perpetrators' responsibility, this new ontology in fact "attenuate[s] the blame game." The "notion of a confederate agency" allows us better to discern broad structural problems and in doing so reveals "individuals as simply incapable of bearing full responsibility" for disasters, diseases, discrimination, and the like deriving from complex underlying interconnections.[9] How might the agency of assemblages help us consider responsibility for irrevocable damage? This, I believe, is the fundamental question with which Hongan no kai member Ogata Masato grapples.

In this chapter, I draw upon Italian philosopher Giorgio Agamben's thought as it engages Primo Levi's account of his lived experience of Auschwitz. In doing so, I do not intend to conflate the experiences of those who suffered in Auschwitz and Minamata. Rather, I extrapolate from Agamben's ethical writings in order to articulate the implicit conceptual framework guiding Ogata's thoughts and actions. I thus employ Agamben's work as a point of reference for understanding Ogata's sometimes enigmatic ethical praxis, which I believe may guide us closer to a world otherwise. Ogata, we will find, reaches the same conclusion as Agamben regarding the impossibility of assuming responsibility for irrevocable damage. Ogata puts into practice what in Agamben's terms is a "new ethical element."

The following pages trace my attempts to understand Ogata's thoughts and actions in order to find practical insights for realizing a world otherwise. As we will see, in his youth, Ogata worked alongside Kawamoto Teruo, leader of the group of Minamata plaintiffs, in bringing their case against Chisso to trial. However, Ogata eventually withdrew from the lawsuit and parted ways with Kawamoto. Given his devotion to the sufferers' movement, Ogata's renunciation of the legal process and removal from the lawsuit surprised both Kawamoto and others involved in the litigation. To better understand Ogata's abrupt withdrawal, this chapter offers a concise biographical overview of Ogata, highlighting the ideas that I believe led to the recognition of a "new ethical element" and corresponding environmental praxis. In doing so, I show that Ogata, like Agamben and Bennett, does not abandon the notion of responsibility, but rather considers it in terms of assemblages. Ogata's ideas and actions commend an ontological shift based upon a new understanding of *ko,* or the individual, which he takes to be always embedded within assemblages. In this way, Ogata's conception of ko thus differs critically from the modern imagination of the individual as independent and autonomous.

AGAMBEN ON ETHICS, LAW, AND RESPONSIBILITY

Calamities such as Minamata pose a challenge for ethicists who grapple with the violence of irreparable injury, in this case damage caused by disposal of a toxic chemical substance, methylmercury. The overarching questions in this chapter for framing the issues and problems to be addressed are as follows: How might ethicists approach situations in which victims die in extreme agony, their bodies out of control, or in which infants experience prenatal exposure to poison? How should we respond when those suffering from such disease have no other means of making a living than exposing themselves to danger, for example, fishing in contaminated waters? And what is the right course of action when victims themselves are blamed for economic decline? How to proceed when the notion of "justice" is called into question by modern systems and structures that give rise to suffering?

Agamben's work offers guidance for such questions of response/responsibility, ethics, and justice. In his book *Remnants of Auschwitz*, Agamben urges readers not to conflate the categories of ethics and law. Agamben cautions against relying on law as the source of moral authority. By Agamben's thinking, "Law is not directed toward the establishment of justice. Nor is it directed toward the verification of truth. Law is solely directed toward judgment, independent of truth and justice."[10] Thus taking law to be concerned with judgment, as separate from truth and justice, Agamben arrives at the following claim: "The ultimate aim of law is the production of a *res judicata* in which the sentence becomes the substitute for the true and the just, being held as true despite its falsity and injustice."[11] Judgments of the law, by Agamben's thinking, do not and cannot realize truth and justice.

If the law produces judgments that counterfeit truth and justice, the punitive and corrective aspects of the law are therefore embedded in the judgments themselves. Agamben cites Italian jurist Sebastiano Satta, who claims that "judgment is itself punishment" and that "the only truly innocent person 'is not the one who is acquitted, but rather the one who goes through life without judgment.'"[12] Even when a defendant is found not guilty, this does not exonerate the defendant from doubt; once one has been suspected as guilty in a legal context, one will never be entirely innocent in the minds of others. Hence, the verdict, guilty or not, functions as punishment. In this way, because law and judgment cannot in fact exert genuine moral authority, they can only ever serve as substitutes of moral authority.

It is for this reason that Agamben separates justice from law; the law pronounces judgments but cannot dispense genuine justice. If justice is separate from law, we must then conceive of justice outside the realm of the law. Agamben believes that if damage is truly irrevocable and irremediable, as in the case in which a person's mind and/or body are permanently harmed, restorative justice under the law necessarily falls short. Consider the damage done to one's fence by a reckless driver. As a result of a legal trial, one might acquire a new, sturdier fence at the expense of the driver (or her insurance company). Replacement might bring some satisfaction, but if the damaged fence carried some emotional value, even a new, sturdier fence will not be satisfactory recompense. When the destruction is irrevocable and the damage is irreparable, any form of legal "justice"— incarceration of the perpetrator, replacement of property, monetary compensation, etc.—is inadequate. This fact does not mean that justice is insignificant. Rather, Agamben's point is that in cases of irremediable harm, we must acknowledge that legal judgments alone will not bring justice, will not repair the damage or harm.

Having analyzed law as distinct from justice, Agamben turns to the task of describing the relation of law to moral responsibility. As his case study, Agamben turns to the 1961 trial of Adolf Eichmann in Jerusalem. At this trial, Eichmann admitted his guilt before God, yet sought to evade legal prosecution, claiming that he was simply obeying the law in carrying out his crimes. Against Eichmann, who dissociated his own moral culpability from legal accountability, Agamben responds: "It must be recalled that the assumption of moral responsibility has value only if one is ready to assume the relevant legal consequences."[13] By this reasoning, "To assume guilt and responsibility—which can, at times, be necessary—is to leave the territory of ethics and enter that of law."[14] This is to say that although law and judicial judgment may be regarded as sources of moral authority, law does not in fact produce moral good; rather, it produces conditions for claiming moral responsibility. As we have seen, we should not, by Agamben's thinking, equate law with morality—but moral responsibility is meaningless without the assumption of legal consequences.

In light of Agamben's reflections on moral responsibility, one may ask whether ethics can address irrevocable damage independent of the law. Ethics, by Agamben's account, is "the doctrine of the happy life"; it concerns neither guilt nor responsibility,[15] which emerge within the purview of the law: "The gesture of assuming responsibility is therefore genuinely juridical and not ethical."[16] Moral responsibility is founded upon legal responsibility, for Agamben, and therefore does not fall into the realm of ethics, separating moral from ethics. While Agamben treats the assumption of legal responsibility as an obligation that everyone must abide, assuming legal responsibility without also claiming moral responsibility "expresses nothing noble or luminous," he writes, "but rather simply obligation."[17]

Having established the distinction between legal and moral responsibilities, it now becomes clear that Agamben's notion of ethics lies beyond both the legal and moral realms. Indeed, Agamben takes ethics to be "before good and evil"; it is a "zone of non-responsibility."[18] But far from indicating a simple lack or eschewal of responsibility, the zone of non-responsibility indicates "confrontation" with the *enormity* of responsibility, a recognition that responsibility exceeds our capability for assuming it. It is "a confrontation with a responsibility that is infinitely greater than any we could ever assume. At the most, we can be faithful to it, that is, assert its unassumability."[19]

In the face of irrevocable damage such as in the case of Minamata, we must admit and dwell with the fact that assuming moral responsibility concomitant with harm is impossible. Admission of the incommensurable enormity of responsibility, Agamben believes, is the only honest and accurate response to irreparable damage, and it is this "irresponsibility" to which ethics addresses itself.[20] Ethics acknowledges moral responsibility, only to make clear the impossibility of assuming it. We can only be "faithful" to it, abide with it.[21] Understood this way, ethics is the domain of thought that identifies the arena in which humans reveal their utter inability to assume responsibility. Agamben's conception of ethics is compatible Edith Wyschogrod's characterization of ethics is "the sphere of transactions between 'self' and 'Other.'"[22] as Wyschogrod asserts, admitting the unassumability of responsibility for the other is, I believe, an ethical act in this sphere.

Following Levi, Agamben invites readers to contemplate a zone in which ethics as traditionally conceived—ethics as the adjudication of good and evil—is preceded by a "zone of irresponsibility." With Levi, he "places ethics before the area in which we are accustomed to consider it."[23] While law is systematized on the distinction between victims and victimizers, in the arena of ethics *before* ethics—the "gray zone," as Primo Levi puts it—the boundary separating victims from victimizers blurs/disappears. Whereas ethics is typically understood as a discourse regarding good and evil, in this gray zone, good and evil are dissolved, "fused." Here "the oppressed becomes oppressor and the executioner in turn appears as victim."[24] This indistinguishability, as we soon will see, is evident in Ogata Masato's thought in the case of Minamata.

In this connection, Agamben's conception of ethics as a zone of non-responsibility may suggestively be brought into conversation with Bennet's notion of the agency of assemblages, in which responsibility does not devolve upon autonomous individuals but is rather "distributed across a mosaic." "In a world of distributed agency," writes Bennett, "a hesitant attitude toward assigning singular blame becomes a presumptive virtue."[25] The hesitancy of which Bennett speaks, I wish to suggest, is something very like dwelling in the zone of non-responsibility. Indeed, Levi and Agamben call attention to forms of systemic violence in which no one is innocent and everyone is culprit—a problem with which Minamata sufferer Ogata also struggles. When lives are damaged or destroyed systematically, any ethics constructed upon the presumption that one is an independent and autonomous being, is inadequate, even irrelevant.

And yet, Agamben finds in the recognition of this inadequacy the possibility of a "new ethical element." In his thought, ethics is "independent of every establishment of [individual] responsibility—one that I believe coincides with a concept of agency as "distributive and confederate," and thus an ethics "detach[ed] from moralism."[26] I wish to show that the task of defining a new ethical element in the zone of irresponsibility *before* ethics was undertaken—though in different terms—by fisher and Minamata sufferer Ogata Masato.

OGATA MASATO: A BIOGRAPHICAL OVERVIEW

The youngest of eighteen siblings, Ogata Masato was born in 1953 on the small peninsula of Meshima, north of Minamata city.[27] Ogata's family business was "fixed shore-net fishing," which eventually "shifted to trawl netting for sardines, and then moved into purse seining,"[28] a move reflecting the modern industrialization of Japan's fishing industry. Ogata was very close to his father, Ogata Fukumatsu, a respected member of Meshima's net-fishing community and one of seven amimoto in the village. In his autobiography, *Tokoyo no fune o kogite: Minamatabyō shishi* (*Rowing the Eternal Sea: The Story of a Minamata Fisherman*), Ogata recounts his idyllic childhood—memories of his father, the fellow fishers working for him, and the abundant gifts of the sea.[29] While Ogata portrays a bucolic fishing life in his early childhood, he also mentions the reality of the community's social hierarchy, in which landowning farmers looked down on landless fishers.[30] Facing such prejudice, Fukumatsu saved enough money to purchase tracts of rice paddy and woodland to provide food for his descendants in case the sea yielded no catch. This property was not the only thing that Ogata inherited from his father. Fukumatsu also influenced Ogata by his very way of life and the value he placed on relations to others—fellow humans, nonhumans, and other-than-humans.

Chapter 3 described the Sugimoto family's conception of their intimate relationship with the fish, the sea, and the natural environment. Fukumatsu likewise developed an idiomatic way of referring to his work as a fisher; he took catching fish to be a "competition" between the spirits of humans and those of fish, thus seeing fish not merely as a resource but as spirited beings closely tied with humans. When Fukumatsu encountered a school of gray mullet in the sea but failed to catch one, he would say, "we lost to the [spirits of the] fish."[31] Such a view extended beyond the creatures of the sea. When dirt was found in the bottom of their boats, the Meshima fishers would say, "the boat's collecting *aka*," using a term for "filth" that applies to humans." When the fishing net was torn, Ogata's father and other fishers would say, "the net has been injured."[32]

Ogata's sense of intimacy with the people, animals, waters, and objects around him was shaken when he was six years old. In 1959, Fukumatsu fell ill, his whole body shaking violently. Ogata's siblings, nephews, and nieces also began to suffer from similar symptoms. The illness would eventually be identified as methylmercury poisoning—Minamata disease. Gradually, the fish began to appear in less abundance, and thus the catches dwindled. At the same time, the market shunned fish from this area, where the kibyō or "strange disease" prevailed. As a result, the fishing business brought in less cash, leading in turn to further discrimination against the fishers, thus reinforcing the prejudicial idea that the kibyō struck only fishers.

Ogata's fishing community, once blessed with abundant harvests, had become a sluggish and stricken. Ogata felt suffocated by his gloomy prospects; the overall health of his family members and the wider community continued to deteriorate while the family fishing business waned. At the age of sixteen, Ogata left his hometown for Kumamoto, the closest urban center, in search of new employment opportunities. Lacking the skills to support himself, however, Ogata became involved with a right-wing *yakuza,* or organized crime group, which often recruited aimless youth lacking resources. Two years later, while he was still a minor, Ogata was arrested while taking part in a demonstration supported by the yakuza. At the correctional center, a counselor informed him that the group he was now affiliated with had in fact supported the Chisso Corporation and even resorted to violence against Minamata sufferers and anti-Chisso activists. This information sobered Ogata, impelling him to leave the yakuza for good. After being released from the correctional center, he severed all ties with the group, fortunately without serious consequences.[33]

Upon returning to his hometown, Ogata became more involved with the Minamata lawsuit, which was led by a well-known local activist, Kawamoto Teruo. After joining the plaintiff's group, Ogata quickly became among the most enthusiastic and dedicated activists. While engaged in activism, he met a group of college students—three male and one female—who had moved to Minamata to support the sufferers. Ogata was intrigued by their motivation for coming to Minamata. Ogata believed that unlike him, the college students had before them the promise of a good life, and could even work for a big corporation like Chisso. Ogata's curiosity led him to befriend and have discussions with the students. These encounters and conversations were to inspire changes to Ogata's thinking.

Thanks to his interactions with these young people, Ogata reflects, "something within me gradually began to awaken. While these students had come to our village with no personal agenda, just to offer their support, I, who had sworn revenge against Chisso, hadn't yet taken a single significant step. I started to ask myself exactly what role I should play (in this struggle)."[34]

This was in 1973, when Minamata was drawing wide public attention, as a new group of sufferers of methylmercury poisoning had been "discovered" in Ariake (following those in Minamata and Niigata prefectures). This revelation disturbed people across Japan.[35] Although the plaintiffs had demanded compensation for all Minamata sufferers, the money was to be distributed only among the *nintei kanja*, or certified patients, approved by the prefectural and national governments.[36]

Witnessing growing divisions among sufferers—who was certified and who was not—Ogata began to feel overwhelmed by doubts about his activism and his own motivations for pursuing it. He was haunted by many questions:

> If I wasn't in the movement for money, was I in it to avenge my father's death? What would happen after I had realized that revenge? Was it just an illusion to entertain the thought that I was putting the interest of others above my own? How could I pretend to be altruistic when I was making my own family suffer (since I devoted myself to the movement)? Did the end justify the means?[37]

Troubled by these questions, he also found himself increasingly frustrated. Despite a long period of negotiations with representatives of the local and central governments and Chisso, Ogata was unable to build relationships with the actual people in charge, who were transferred from one office to another every few years. Coming from a world that valued relationships among people and with the environment, Ogata found such impersonal interactions at court not only meaningless but unbearable. Furthering his disappointment, the negotiations always ultimately revolved around money—calculations of the worth of human lives. Unable to continue with the process, Ogata disengaged from the movement and withdrew from the lawsuit.

By Ogata's reckoning, the legal battles had the consequence of depersonalizing individual suffering. Precisely because of the "fairness" that the law demanded, discussions in court had to be objective, impartial, and therefore inevitably impersonal. The nature of the law prevented Ogata from building relationships with government officials or Chisso workers, as he had always done with beings around him. Instead, the system only permitted him to confront the defendants' representatives.

What Ogata sought—and what the lawsuit could not accomplish—was to address the Minamata sufferers' physical pains as well as their emotional distress from discrimination. Above all, Ogata was troubled by the Chisso defendants' indifference to the sufferers' plight, severed from their fellow fishers and natural surroundings. Ogata repeatedly felt betrayed by the court, which treated as insignificant their demands to redress the violence that upended their lives in so many ways—not simply the agony from the illness, but the broken relations with their neighbors and even the creatures in the sea. Ogata's goal was to reestablish and foster relations among and between humans and their surroundings. Failure to achieve this goal would amount to a miscarriage of justice. The court's exclusive focus on monetary compensation was therefore entirely dissatisfying. The final blow in Ogata's inner struggle was the fact that, as he acknowledged, the sufferers' movement had itself become increasingly bureaucratic and faceless, coming to resemble the governments and Chisso. He expressed his disappointment that the movement "had shifted from the streets to the court."[38]

He described his discomfort with the movement: "It seemed that no one wanted to address the more important issues. But the problem was that not even I could clearly identify those issues."[39] The Chisso Corporation was surely culpable, having discharged methylmercury for a period of nearly three decades even after suspicion had been raised; the prefectural and central governments were also guilty, having turned a blind eye to Chisso's misconduct in order to preserve corporate profits and economic stability in and beyond Minamata. Ogata was discouraged that the court was not interested in discussing how to change the system that had given rise to the disease. Here we may recall Agamben: the law functions only to produce judgments, not justice. While the civil court's decision found Chisso accountable for the disease and ordered compensation to the sufferers, Ogata's vision of justice—the restoration of relationships among and between humans and their surroundings—remained unaddressed in court.

Viewing Minamata disease and its aftermath as systemic problems, Ogata was convinced that the legal responsibility assigned to Chisso, as well as both the local and central governments, failed to address the holistic restoration of what had been lost. Ogata's foremost concern was to reconstitute humans' relations to each other and to their surroundings—what had truly been lost. Restoration of such relations would require an ontological shift of a sort that could hardly be addressed in a legal context.[40] Ogata consequently reached a conclusion that resonates with Agamben's claim about responsibility: "The idea of assuming responsibility," Ogata writes, "is an illusion. Our legal proceedings are premised on this illusion. We make the assumption that, if we pay reparations, we have assumed responsibility."[41] Ogata's provocative statement amounts to a challenge to the foundation of the modern judiciary.

Like Agamben, Ogata believes the assumption of responsibility for irreparable damage to be ultimately impossible. But these thinkers acknowledge that we must nevertheless assume "relevant legal consequences," for the "gesture of assuming a juridical responsibility" is what gives "value" to the "assumption of moral responsibility"[42] This point is borne out in Chisso president Shimada Ken'ichi's meeting with Kawamoto Teruo. Shimada, who assumed the presidency of Chisso in 1971, had occasion to meet face to face with the Minamata sufferers. Facing Shimada, Kawamoto challenged him: "You once said, 'If they [Minamata sufferers] hold a grudge, it must be against me. I will take all the responsibility,' didn't you?" To this inquire, Shimada replied:

> That was not my intention. What I meant was that a company is where employees are hired to work [not to make decisions]. In this regard, they are not held accountable [for the company's wrongdoings]. That is why I said that I was responsible for what had happened. I assure you that I would not mind a trial and the relevant sentence, but let the employees go as unpunished. My memory serves that this is what I stated.[43]

Shimada thus acknowledges his own responsibility as a decision-making executive (and he was perhaps one of the most conscientious executives at the time). But Shimada's seemingly "noble" willingness to assume juridical responsibility on behalf of Chisso employees remains in the realm of law. It therefore "expresses nothing noble or luminous, but rather simply obligation."[44] He is utterly incapable of assuming responsibility for the death and suffering caused by Chisso's pollution, unable to restore a "normal" life to the people of Minamata. Such pleas are beyond restorative justice in the sphere of the law.

Tsuchimoto Noriaki's documentary film *Minamata* poignantly conveys the irrevocable damage of the disease and the utter incapability of individuals like Shimada to take responsibility for it.[45] But it also provokes the question, germane to our discussion of responsibility, of whether Shimada, too, is a victim of the modern system of which he is a part. I hardly wish to suggest that the Chisso president's difficulties to the plight of Minamata sufferers, which are incommensurable. That said, the documentary demonstrates that Shimada was a "cog" in the corporate machinery, someone who happened to be in the president position during the case against Chisso. (Shimada was aware of what he was entering into when he assumed the position.) Being a "cog" by no means exonerates Shimada from the crimes perpetrated by the corporation which he served, but the observation does lead us to see that "Chisso"—itself an impersonal corporate system—epitomizes the other systems in our society.

The investigation also discloses the complex relations between and among victims and victimizers. The documentary *Minamata* shows with distressing clarity the zone of non-responsibility, showing that none could take responsibility for the lost lives, impaired health, and damaged environment and likewise revealing the zone of irresponsibility. There, the very system that imposed and reinforced the concept of good and evil, in fact, nullifies the boundaries of good and evil by depriving humans of their agency—a kind of agency upon which the system is founded. Ogata witnessed all these complications, too.

LEAVING THE MOVEMENT, WITHDRAWING FROM THE LAWSUIT

Ogata describes the period during which he distanced himself from the movement—a *kurui,* or a phase of insanity, in which he experienced guilt, frustration, and a loss of self-identity. During this time, he pondered what he could have done differently, had he been a Chisso employee. What would he have done when the factory was thriving and the city was not only benefiting from it but indeed dependent on it? Ogata wondered whether he might have raised his voice on behalf of those dying from the contaminated wastewater. Or what if, at sixteen years of age, Ogata had found a job opportunity at the Chisso factory? Rather than flee to Kumamoto city, he might have taken employment with the company. Were he to have become a whistleblower, it would have meant the loss of his job, and therefore not only the loss of a stable income but also any other job prospects in Minamata, where he would have been seen as a traitor.[46] Even worse, he thought, the consequences of whistleblowing would likely have extended to members of his family, who would have been socially ostracized or bullied at school.[47] For many reasons, then, leveling a public accusation against Chisso would have had serious social repercussions. Pondering these scenarios, Ogata found it difficult to blame the Chisso workers who had denied and dismissed the sufferers' claims.[48]

It was with this new perspective that Ogata arrived at a crucial realization; he recognized himself as one of *them*: *Chisso wa watashi de atta* ("I have become another Chisso," or "Chisso within"). The realization makes clear that the entire system was what Levi referred to as a "gray zone" in which the "'long chain of conjunction between victim and executioner' comes loose, where the oppressed becomes oppressor and the executioner in turn appears as victim."[49] Or in Ogata's own words, "What Chisso represented is a question we must ask ourselves today. This may sound strange, but I think that Chisso might have been another me, myself."[50] Realizing that Chisso represented only a larger system whose values Ogata himself internalized and literally embodied, he continued his confession:

> For the past forty years, I have owned a car, a TV set, a refrigerator, and a plastic-based fishing boat. In other words, I am surrounded by so many things made at chemical factories like Chisso. For example, most of the polyvinyl chloride used for the faucets at home was made at Chisso, or a more recent example of a Chisso product is the liquid crystal used for computers and TV screens. We live surrounded by Chisso products. If we talk only about the Minamata incident, the Chisso Corporation is responsible for it, but in this present time, we all have already become "another Chisso." The society that has pursued modernization and affluence has become ourselves.[51]

By consuming those products, even the sufferers of methylmercury poisoning—most likely unconsciously—take part in sustaining Chisso, the very entity that destroyed their health, the lives of their loved ones, their livelihoods, and their community. In the face of these relations with Chisso, Ogata confessed his own complicity: "[When at trial] Chisso is the Other, the enemy, the assailant. For me, however, this viewpoint evolved until I recognized 'The Chisso within.'"[52]

The realization that he was a victim harboring the victimizer within placed Ogata in the gray zone (Levi) or zone of irresponsibility (Agamben).[53] Agamben believes that the cruelty of Auschwitz not only obscures the demarcation line separating victims from victimizers but also renders pointless the distinction between life and death, good and evil, and humans and nonhumans, as the ethical resources for sorting out one's moral authority are long exhausted. However, this seemingly gloomy picture might indicate the illusion of independent and autonomous human agency.

Under such circumstances, Ogata embarked on the task of learning how to navigate the gray zone, where existing categories would not help. Though he decided to withdraw from the lawsuit and consequently forfeit any compensation from Chisso, he refrained from condemning those who continued to pursue the lawsuit and accept the payouts. But some sufferers and their supporters criticized Ogata on the grounds that his withdrawal made it difficult for others to receive compensation, that his departure undermined the solidarity of the citizens' movement, or that he was merely seeking public recognition. Yet others accused Ogata of giving the governments and the corporation an easy way out by not insisting on their legal responsibility. I understand the concern that Ogata's withdrawal would potentially weaken the movement, and I generally would not endorse this tactic in other situations. As the Complainants demonstrated after the Fukushima nuclear meltdown, their trail against TEPCO CEOs enabled the plaintiffs to gather and submit a large volume of evidence, otherwise dispersed or undisclosed. In Ogata's case, in my sympathetic reading, I do see his gesture as a sincere attempt to seek an alternative outside the legal system for imputing responsibility.

First, Ogata himself emphasized that his decision should not be taken to pressure those who were suffering financially, and thus in need of the payout. Leaving the court case was, for him, an expression of determination to seek an alternative to the modern legal system, yet it does not suggest that he found the litigation efforts meaningless. Like Agamben, he believes in the "necessity of the trials . . . despite their evident insufficiency."[54] For not only do trials have a socially pragmatic value (the Minamata case served to disseminate information about the disease and plight of the sufferers); it also reveals the limits of the law, forcing "confrontation with a responsibility infinitely greater than any we could ever assume."[55] Viewed from Ogata and

Agamben's perspective, the trial in fact compels us to hesitate before assigning blame. Recognizing the inadequacy of the law obliges us to dwell in the zone of non-responsibility.

For Ogata, this hesitation, this entry into the "gray zone," was itself not without considerable cost to his well-being. Ogata found himself falling into a state of kurui before finally finding a way out, leading toward a world otherwise. Ogata emphasized that his withdrawal from the lawsuit should remind the state and the corporation that he "did not forgive the authorities" and did not abide by their rules.[56] "There are," says Ogata, "still people [like me] who, as long as they live, will never say, 'It's over.' These people cannot be judged by the standards of the Establishment. The system is at a loss as to how to deal with them."[57] Thus, his withdrawal from the trial and movement by no means signified resignation; refusing the rules that govern the establishment, Ogata embodies the possibility of a world otherwise.

Ogata's denial of the state's authority and corporate power may be better understood in light of Herman Melville's depiction of Bartleby in his 1853 story "Bartleby, the Scrivener: A Story of Wall Street." In this story, an elderly narrator recounts the curious ways of the titular character. The plot concerns a lawyer who has two petulant scriveners, Nippers and Turkey, in his employ, and who decides to hire a third scrivener in the hope that his more placid demeanor might mitigate the tension between the other two. Upon hire, Bartleby proves to be highly productive. One day, however, when asked to proofread a document, Bartleby declines the request with the phrase that will become his refrain: "I would prefer not to." From this point, Bartleby produces less and less, eventually ceasing work entirely. He then begins to live out of the office. His employer makes a few attempts to talk him out of his "irrational" behavior but to no avail. Despite his employer's efforts, Bartleby continues to stay in the office, producing no work until he is forcibly removed and thrown into jail. In the end, he dies of hunger, as he "preferred not to" eat. The narrator then discovers that Bartleby had once worked at a dead-letter office, and he attributes the scrivener's behavior to this previous job.

Melville's story is enigmatic. At first glance, the narrative may not seem to offer much help toward formulating viable modes of refusal; after all, the death of the protagonist may suggest he has been defeated. Philosopher Slavoj Žižek, however, reads the story as opening up a space exterior to the politics of resistance—one that resonates with Ogata's withdrawal from the lawsuit:

> In his refusal of the Master's order, Bartleby does not negate the predicate; rather, he affirms a non-predicate: he does not say that he *doesn't want to do it;* he says that *he prefers (wants) not to do it.* This is how we pass from the politics of "resistance" or "protestation," which parasitizes upon what it negates,

to a politics which opens up a new space outside the hegemonic position and its negation.[58]

If Bartleby's reply had been "I don't want to do it," then he would simply be refusing the order, and his refusal would thereby demonstrate recognition of the authority, verifying its power. By responding, "I would prefer not to," however, Bartleby reframes the relations between his employer and himself, asserting his exteriority to the "existing universe of social machinery."

In light of Žižek's interpretation of Bartleby, we may now see that Ogata's withdrawal is neither a sign of resignation nor the mark of subjugation to authority. On the contrary, it demonstrates a genuine subversiveness, for, in withdrawing, Ogata accedes to a position outside the modern system of law and power. Ogata's refusal to continue negotiations with Chisso on their turf, his refusal of compensation money from Chisso doled out to those who had been officially certified as "patients," recalls Bartleby's refrain; with his actions, Ogata symbolically says, "I prefer not to." Ogata's actions, at once beyond the prevailing social and legal order and its hierarchies, and yet firmly embedded in a reality of human sufferings and relations, gestures toward a world otherwise.

ONTOLOGICAL SHIFT: *TAMASHII* (SPIRIT) AND *KO* (INDIVIDUALS)

The worldview on which Ogata relied on withdrawing from the legal procedure was one he inherited from his father and fellow fishers. In their world, nurturing and refining tamashii, or the spirit, was valued above all else. It is a life force, "the very core of existence."[59] In fact, the title of Hongan no kai's newsletter, *Tamashii utsure*, "Transferring the spirit," came from one of Ogata's favorite childhood memories, in which his father, Fukumatsu, put his forehead against Ogata's and said "tamashii utsure." With this gesture, Fukumatsu passed knowledge, affection, and values to a person for whom he cared—a way of acknowledging the tamashii innate in every being and transferring "the memory of life" (Figure 4.1).[60]

Tamashii, Ogata observes, "is found even in non-organic beings that humans created, such as tools and objects."[61] Tamashii dwells not only in human beings but in fishing tools and appliances. One might recall that a boat has funadama (the spirit of a boat), which is venerated by fishers. Tamashii facilitates communications among beings, whether human or not. Thus, when Ogata tried to build relationships with Chisso, he was frustrated not only because he could not find any tamashii in the Chisso executives but also because the court a place from which tamashii are excluded. Ogata relies on tamashii to articulate the reasoning behind his withdrawal from the lawsuit: "I

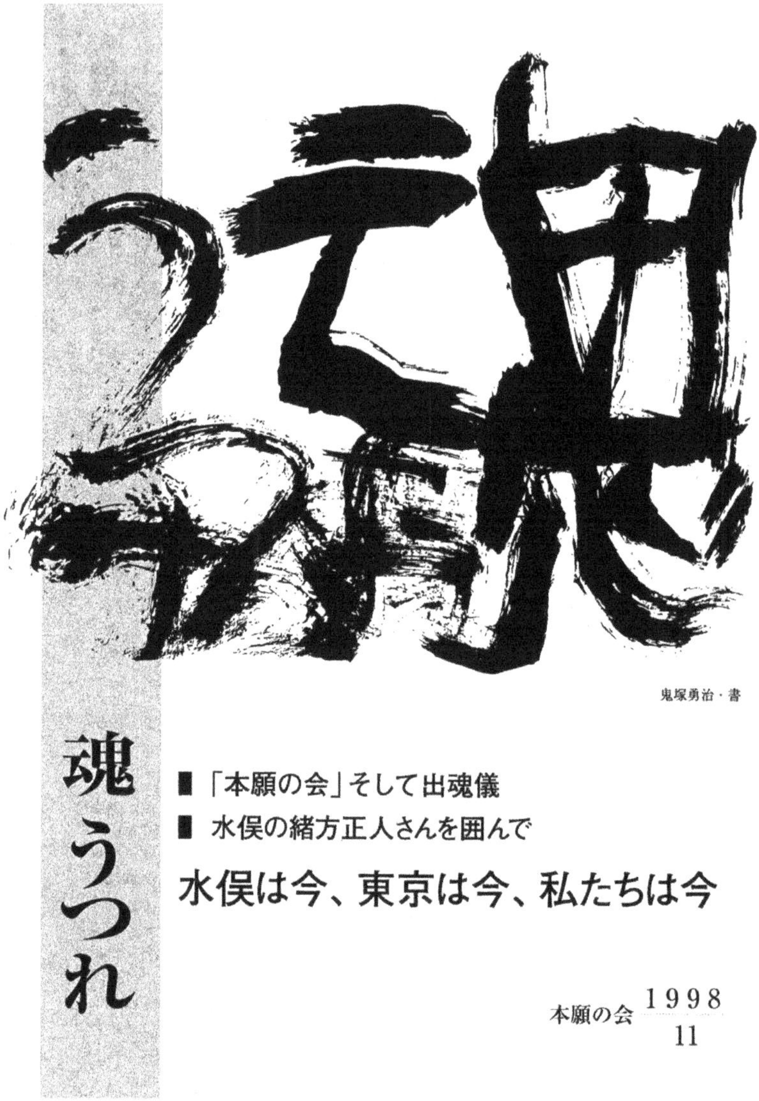

Figure 4.1 The Cover Page of the First Issue of *Tamashii utsure*. 1998.

think that the problem [emerging out of Minamata] that cannot be addressed by politics is a very fundamental and essential problem. That is, the problems cannot be resolved by policies and systems but concern our tamashii."[62]

Tamashii is not simply a value-neutral core of a being; rather, as people of Minamata believe, it concerns moral character: a person who is dishonest or unkind is described as a *tamashii no asaka* fellow, or a person with a shallow spirit, while a person who is honest and compassionate is referred to as a *tamashii no fukaka* one, or a person whose spirit is profound. Ogata, playing with the word, encapsulates the essence of tamashii: "When our tamashii gets *nigoru* (muddy or turbid), it becomes *damashii*, or deception. The best example is found in the history of Japan: when the military controlled the nation, Japan invaded other countries under the banner of *yamato damashii* (Japanese spirit/deception). We must not forget that the muddy spirit like yamato damashii deceived and brainwashed people."[63] When tamashii gets lost or becomes shallow, believes Ogata, one is easily appropriated by the system, becoming a "cog"—a condition leading to loss of contact with one's tamashii.

Given this understanding of tamashii, one begins to see that what Chisso destroyed was not only the Minamata people's lives, health, environment, and community but also, at a more profound level, humans' relations to tamashii. This includes the stories and moral traits shared generally by people in Minamata through tamashii. Retrieving tamashii, according to Ogata, means restoring the world and our relations to ourselves, to nonhumans, and other-than-humans. He thus observes, "My life comes into being in this continuation of others' lives."[64] That is why catching fish is sacred; it is a communication with the fish through tamashii. Tamashii is a vessel of life force and a vehicle of memory.

However, the perception of tamashii as innate in each entity may sound similar to the idea of modern agency, with its presumption of independence and autonomy. In the 2004 newsletter of *Tamashii utsure*, Ogata engaged in a dialogue with sociologist Kurihara Akira, clarifying the notion of tamashii in relation to the Japanese term *ko*. Ko is conventionally translated in English as "individuals," but Kurihara explains that *ko* "is not so-called individualism. I am not talking about the individual who is atomized, quantified, and at last becomes a piece of information, but about an individual who is open to life-force (*seimei sonzai*)."[65] The life force, Ogata explains, is a function of life (*inochi no hataraki*), but life here is not restricted to sentient beings but extends to nonorganic beings, nonhumans, and other-than-humans. Indeed, Ogata believes even the dead can influence our present lives through their life-force.

Ogata's construal of ko suggests a way to reconceptualize ontology and reconfigure being, not as closed and autonomous agencies, but as open to communication with all possible beings—an idea that resonates with Bennett's notion of the agency of assemblages. Bennett is not the only thinker who calls for such an ontological shift: Stephen K. White's "weak ontology" (which takes a nonfoundationalist position inspired by the works by Charles Taylor)[66] and Judith Butler's "thin ontology," among others, recognize how traditional Western ontologies asserting the primacy of the autonomous individual are implicated in war, economic inequities, environmental depredations, and other malaises associated with modernity.

Among the theories advocated by these acclaimed thinkers, Bennett's resonates most closely with Ogata's ontology——not "thin" or "weak," but diffusive, spreading out, forming assemblages across the boundaries of this world and beyond, unconfined by time and space. Furthermore, Bennett's concept of the agency of assemblages is, as we have already noted, compatible with the theories of Agamben. Bennett asserts that a new ontology of the agency of assemblages will help reshape the notion of ethics: "An understanding of agency as distributive and confederate thus reinvokes the need to detach ethics from moralism and to produce guides to action appropriate to a world of vital, crosscutting forces."[67] Bennett thus urges readers to consider that "perhaps the ethical responsibility of an individual human now resides in one's response to the assemblages in which one finds oneself participating."[68]

Oagata's reconception of the "individual" as ko, that is, as always embedded within assemblages, may constitute a new ethical element. Condoning a vision of a world inhabited by ko, Ogata also calls for awareness that each individual is anchored by tamashii, unconstrained by the boundaries of this present world. His notion of ko promotes an ontology of the agency of assemblages, which may in turn give rise to a "new ethical element." Bennett emphasizes that what distinguishes between the perception of oneself as a part of the agency of assemblages and a cog in a machine lies in one's response to the confederated entity of which one is a part—a corporation, a fisher's cooperative, a nation-state, or what have you. In order for this ontology to constitute a new ethical element, she urges her readers to ask themselves: "Do I attempt to extricate myself from assemblages whose trajectory is likely to do harm?" and "Do I enter into the proximity of assemblages whose conglomerate effectivity tends toward the enactment of nobler ends?"[69]

It is critical to understand that assemblages do not always align with the categorical boundaries that prevail in our modern world; one may therefore find oneself unexpectedly in an assemblage that one had not previously recognized as existing or even as possible. An openness and willingness to form assemblages is the new ethical element. Therefore, holding onto the idea of tamashii, ko, and the agency of assemblages requires us a willingness to dwell in ambiguity and uncertainty, to partake of something like what poet John Keats called "negative capability"—the ability to remain in a state of perpetual and perceptual openness to "vital, crosscutting forces"[70] One need not, and indeed cannot, abandon this world in becoming part of a world otherwise.[71] As Ogata and Bennett make clear, the notion of a world otherwise is an ever-renewed possibility for transforming the modern world.

In fact, many in this world experience transactions between the two worlds, for example, when speaking at the grave of a loved one. Ogata points to examples of such transactions observable in Japan, such as the *obon*, a belief in which people welcome dead spirits returning to this world. This belief is often associated with Buddhism, though it contradicts the Buddhist principle of reincarnation.[72] Ogata describes this connection between the two worlds—separated neither chronologically nor spatially: "We fishers," says Ogata, "live thanks to the fish. We are indebted for our lives to the sea, where we will return upon our death."[73] The world to which he will return does not exist independently from this world; rather, the spirit that remains after bodily death will exist in this world, mingling among the fish. This cosmology, ontology, and ethics constitute a world otherwise. Yet, not many of this world have special relationships with their natural surroundings, such as the fish and the sea. The next two chapters will guide readers to explore this world otherwise, and instruct a way to traffic the two worlds in reading Ishimure's literature.

NOTES

1. Daisuke Kikuchi, "In First, Government and TEPCO Found Liable for Fukushima Disaster," *The Japan Times,* March 17, 2017. http://www.japantimes.co.jp/news/2017/03/17/national/crime-legal/first-government-tepco-found-liable-fukushima-disaster/#.WUrEe_qrpp8.
2. "Fukushima Nuke Disaster Evacuees Disappointed by Court's Compensation Award," *Mainichi shimbun,* March 18, 2017.
3. "Fukushima Nuke Disaster Evacuees Disappointed by Court's Compensation Award." For clarification on the class-action suit, refer to note 3 by Norma Field, "From Fukushima: To Despair Properly, To Find the Next Step," *The Asia-Pacific Journal* 14, no. 17 (3) (2016). https://apjjf.org/2016/17/Field.html.
4. Field, "From Fukushima."
5. As of July 2020, the Complainants appealed the case to a higher court.
6. Eiji Shimura, "Ex-TEPCO Execs Plead Innocent over Fukushima Nuclear Disaster," *The Asahi Shimbun*, June 30, 2017.
7. Shimura, "Ex-TEPCO Execs Plead Innocent over Fukushima Nuclear Disaster."
8. For example, Urlick Beck states, "In the risk society the unknown and unintended consequences come to be a dominant force in history and society" and the risk is distributed more and more unevenly. Urlick Beck, *Risk Society: Towards a New Modernity* (New York: Sage Publications, 1992), 22.
9. Bennett, *Vibrant Matter*, 37.
10. Giorgio Agamben, *Remnants of Auschwitz: The Witness and the Archive*, trans. Daniel Hellier-Roazen (New York: Zone Books, 2002), 18.
11. Agamben, *Remnants of Auschwitz*: 18.
12. Agamben, *Remnants of Auschwitz*, 19, citing Satta 1994. Michel Foucault also refers to punishment: "We must first rid ourselves of the illusion that penalty is

above all (if not exclusively) a means of reducing crime and that, in this role, according to the social forms, the political systems or beliefs, it may be severe or lenient, tend towards expiation of obtaining redress, towards the pursuit of individuals or the attribution of collective responsibility. We must analyse rather the 'concrete systems of punishment,' study them as social phenomena that cannot be accounted for by the juridical structure of society alone, nor by its fundamental ethical choices." Michel Foucault, *Discipline and Punish: The Birth of the Prison*, trans. by Alan Scheridan (New York: Vintage Books, 1977), 24.

13. Agamben, *Remnants of Auschwitz*, 23. Albert Camus points to the issue of acknowledgment of one's culpability. "All I ask is that, in the midst of a murderous world, we agree to reflect on murder and to make a choice. After that, we can distinguish those who accept the consequences of being murderers themselves or the accomplices of murders, and those who refuse to do so with all their force and being." Albert Camus, *Neither Victims nor Executioners: An Ethic Superior to Murder* (Eugene, OR: Wipf & Stock, 2007 [1946]), 55.

14. Agamben, *Remnants of Auschwitz*, 24.

15. Agamben, *Remnants of Auschwitz*, 24.

16. Agamben, *Remnants of Auschwitz*, 22.

17. Agamben, *Remnants of Auschwitz*, 22.

18. Agamben, *Remnants of Auschwitz*, 21.

19. Agamben, *Remnants of Auschwitz*, 21.

20. Agamben, *Remnants of Auschwitz*, 21.

21. Agamben, *Remnants of Auschwitz*, 21.

22. Edith Wyschogrod, *Saints and Postmodernism: Revisioning Moral Philosophy* (Chicago: University of Chicago Press, 1990), xv.

23. Agamben, *Remnants of Auschwitz*, 21.

24. Agamben, *Remnants of Auschwitz*, 21.

25. Bennett, *Vibrant Matter*, 38.

26. Agamben, *Remnants of Auschwitz*, 21.

27. Ogata, *Rowing the Eternal Sea*, 25. When counting two additional children that his mother had before she married Ogata's father, Ogata is the youngest of twenty siblings.

28. Ogata, *Rowing the Eternal Sea*, 26.

29. As chapter 3 reveals, the Chisso factory in Minamata had already negatively affected the environment in the 1920s, but the destruction was then limited to the nearby area and did not affect Meshima, where the Ogata family lived.

30. The elevated status of rice farmers, in contrast to the poor image of non-farmers and non-landowners, has been contested as being a modern construction by many historians, such as Amino Yoshihiko and Tanaka Akihiko, to name only two. Even though non-farmers and nonlandowners were far from poor in certain areas, however, the ideology was firmly rooted in people's mind and was internalized among farmers as well as non-farmers, leading to Fukumatsu's purchase of a piece of land.

31. Ogata, *Rowing the Eternal Sea*, 3–5. Although Karen Colligan-Taylor translates *tamashii kurabe* as "competing souls," I use the translation of "competing spirits."

32. Ogata, *Rowing the Eternal Sea*, 35.

33. Ogata, *Rowing the Eternal Sea*, 69–70. Leaving the organized crime group sometimes required one to cut off one's little finger as a token of apology. In Ogata's case, he was able to leave the group rather amicably.

34. Ogata, *Rowing the Eternal Sea,* 77.

35. Watanabe, Shin'ichi and Seki, Reiko, "'Dai-san Minamatabyō' mondai no genzaiteki isou I: 'Dai-san Minamatabyō' to suigin panikku" (The problem of "the third outbreak of Minamata disease" and its present implications I: "The third outbreak of Minamata disease" and mercury panic), *Oitakenritsu geijutsubunka tankidaigaku kenkyū kiyō* 33 (1995), 48–49. However, the following year, the Environmental Agency concluded that there was no third outbreak of Minamata disease. Ibid., 55–57.

36. Even then, the compensation was divided into three different categories, depending upon the sufferers' symptoms.

37. Ogata, *Rowing the Eternal Sea,* 92.

38. Ogata, *Rowing the Eternal Sea,* 88.

39. Ogata, *Rowing the Eternal Sea,* 92.

40. Ogata, *Rowing the Eternal Sea*, 42–43. Translation mine.

41. Ogata, Masato, *Chisso wa watashi de atta* (I have become another Chisso) (Fukuoka: Ashi shobō, 2001), 145.

42. Agamben, *Remnants of Auschwitz*, 23.

43. Minamatabyō jishu kōshō Kawamoto saiban shiryōshū (Minamata disease direct negotiation group, Kamaoto trial documents) (Tokyo: Gendai jānarizumu shuppankai, 1981), 455.

44. Agamben, *Remnants of Auschwitz*, 22.

45. Tsuchimoto, Noriaki, *Minamata: Kanja san to sono sekai* (Minamata: The victims and their world) 1971.

46. According to the *Report on Minamata Disease 2001*, citing the *Minamata kōjō shimbun* (Chisso Minamata plant news), "The sum of the municipal property tax of the Minamata plant and the municipal tax of its employees exceeded 50% of the income from municipal rates in around 1955, and Chisso must be the first consideration for Minamata, as Chisso is just a money-maker for Minamata City." *Report on Minamata Disease 2001*, 11–12.

47. "In 1960, employees of Chisso and the subcontractor companies accounted for 4,757 (c. 24%) of the industrial population 15 years of age or over (19,819)." *Report on Minamata Disease 2001*, 11.

48. Ogata, *Chisso wa watashi de atta*, 44.

49. Agamben, *Remnants of Auschwitz*, 21.

50. Ogata, *Chisso wa watashi de atta*, 49. The translation is from Yoneyama, "Life-World," 9.

51. Ogata, *Chisso wa watashi de atta,* 49. Translation mine.

52. Ogata, *Rowing the Eternal Sea*, 146.

53. Agamben, *Remnants of Auschwitz*, 21.

54. Agamben, *Remnants of Auschwitz,* 19.

55. Agamben, *Remnants of Auschwitz,* 21.

56. Ogata, *Rowing the Eternal Sea*, 155.
57. Ogata, *Rowing the Eternal Sea*, 155–156.
58. Slavoj Žižek, *The Parallax View* (Cambridge; MA: MIT Press, 2006), 382–383.
59. Sōshisha newsletter, *Gonzui*. 83 (2004): 3.
60. *Gonzui*, 83 (2004): 3.
61. *Gonzui*, 83 (2004): 3.
62. Ogata, Masato, "Tamashii no yukue" (Whereabouts of the spirit), *Tamashii utsure* 1 (1998): 17.
63. Ogata, Masato, "Jikū o koete tobeyo tamashii" (*Tamashii:* Fly beyond the time), *Tamashii utsure* 4 (2001): 3.
64. Ogata, Masato, "Watashitachi wa nani o shiteirunodarou, soshite doko e ikitainodarou" (What are we doing, and where do we want to go?), *Tamashii utsure* 54 (2013): 21.
65. Ogata, Masato and Kurihara, Akira, "Shinsaku Noh ni takusu mono—naze ima hōnō ka" (What we entrust in a new noh play: Why noh now?), *Tamashii utsure* 18 (2004): 17–18.
66. White defines *weak ontology* as follows: "Weak ontology is concerned with the constitution of, and reflection upon, the basic figures of portrayals that animate our thought and action." Stephen K. White, "Weak Ontology: Genealogy and Critical Issues," *Hedgehog Review*, 7, no. 2 (2005): 13. Also see Stephen K. White, "As the World Turns: Ontology and Politics in Judith Butler," *Polity* 32, no. 2 (1999).
67. Bennett, *Vibrant Matter,* 38.
68. Bennett, *Vibrant Matter,* 37.
69. Bennett, *Vibrant Matter,* 37–38.
70. Bennett, *Vibrant Matter*, 38. See also p. 14: "The ethical task at hand here is to cultivate the ability to discern nonhuman vitality, to become perceptually open to it."
71. Ogata, Masato, "Kichou kouen 'souseiki o mukaeta Minamata' seimei kyōdōtai no jichi kaifuku shiyou" ("Keynote speech 'Minamata at the Genesis' Restore the sovereignty of a life-community"), *Tamashii utsure* 29 (2007): 5.
72. Ogata, Masato, "Intabyū: Hontō no kuni o motomete" (Interview: Seeking for the true home), *Gonzui* 94 (2006): 3.
73. Ogata, Masato, "Sakana ya tori ni dou wabirunoka" (How can we apologize to fishes and birds?), *Tamashii tusure* 3 (2000): 13.

Chapter 5

Literature of Dystopia

Ishimure Michiko and the Fragile Power of the Precariousness

RELIGULOUS, RELIGION, RELIGIOSITY

In the 2008 documentary *Religulous*, Bill Maher interviews people about their religious beliefs—primarily rather extreme ones.[1] Over the course of the film, Maher elaborates upon his interpretation of "religion," which he equates with blind faith. He even characterizes those who consider themselves moderately religious to be "enablers" or "mafia wives." His attitude toward religion is conditioned by a post-Enlightenment Protestant Christian framework, where the central components of religion are faith and/or belief.[2] In the final chapter of the movie, Maher continues to insist that religious people are "irrational," whereas atheists (or agnostics) exhibit a rational skepticism regarding matters of religious belief. Then, for his parting shot, Maher admonishes religious believers to "grow up," urging them to abandon their beliefs, which he takes to be at best immature and worst quasi-criminal in their implications. Maher narrates his plea against background of violent and horrific images—from the city of Hiroshima being obliterated by the atomic bomb to the mushroom cloud emerging at a nuclear test site, from the combat training of a (seemingly) paramilitary group to a seabird covered with oil spilled into the ocean and to a glacier disintegrating from global warming.

Religulous gives rise to two issues that concern me here: the first is Maher's reductive equation of religion and irrationality; the second, stemming from the first, is his insistence that religion (divorced from rationality) too often espouses violence. Regarding my first concern, voluminous scholarship refutes the simplistic equation of religion with "blind" faith or belief alone, treating myriad modes of religious expression. Such oversimplifications as Maher's are not merely inadequate, but sometimes harmful.

Consider, for example, the Danish cartoon controversy of 2005, in which Danish newspaper, *Jylands-Posten* published twelve cartoons, mocking the prophet's figures and Islamic faith for its September 30 issue in 2005. Those images soon provoked demonstrations beyond Danish borders, calling for hundreds of thousands of protesters, resulted in "nearly 250 dead and 800 or so wounded."[3] Reflecting this controversy and the discourse brought forth from it, religious studies scholar Saba Mahmood painstakingly reveals the arbitrariness of the binary division of the "religious" and the "secular" that was widely applied in discourse around this controversy.[4] Mahmood argues that relations with "icons" in the Islamic faith are constituted and practiced in a manner that bespeaks an "intimacy with the prophet" Muhammed, one in which the icon is not merely a "referential sign," as in Christian iconographic relations, but rather one of "immanence." In Muslim piety, the "modality of attachment . . . between a devout Muslim and the exemplary figure of Muhammed" is one of "embodied habitation and intimate proximity."[5] In Christianity, meanwhile, the signifier of the icon is not ontologically coextensive with its divine signified; the framework of relationality is therefore quite different. Failing to take into consideration such differences, many commentators framed the cartoon controversy in reductive terms of the secular "liberal value of freedom of speech" vs. "religious taboo," which eventually "crystallized [in] the sense that it was a clash between secular liberal values and an irascible religiosity." Mahmood challenges this reductive framework, seeking to "unsettle" the "consensus across opposed camps,"[6] revealing the "normative understanding of religion internal to liberalism."[7]

Mahmood also calls readers' attention to the fact that the European Court of Human Rights (ECHR) presumes this normative understanding of religion, which includes seeing religion as "fundamentally a matter of choice,"[8] thereby "moral injury" done due to religious identities is not taken seriously, unlike harms because of gender and sexual orientations. As Mahmood observes, framing religion as a choice is itself rooted in the Protestant Christian tradition that upholds the post-Enlightenment conception of the person as an autonomous agent. The ECHR's implicit conception of religion, yet, manifests in preferential decisions favoring protection of "Christian sensibilities" against that which they deem "offensive."[9] While religion is rendered a personal choice, the decisions of the ECHR that valuing Christian sensibilities reveals its contradicting attitude toward religion—the discussion we will revisit in chapter 7.

The second concern I wish to address is that associating religion with irrationality and violence distracts attention from state-sponsored and profit-driven violence.[10] For example, Maher's film, as noted above, contains images of nuclear explosions. Recognizing the danger posed by the prospect of such weaponry falling into the hands of a religious (and thus irrational) "terrorist" group eschews the fact that the only entities that have actually detonated nuclear arms—whether in conflict, tests, or accidents—are mostly "secular" nation-states (the United States, the USSR, France, United Kingdom, China,

India, Pakistan, and North Korea), not a religiously motivated group. Moreover, those "rational" nation-states have conducted over 2,000 nuclear tests altogether—atmospheric, underground, and underwater.[11] This excessive testing and consequent environmental destruction are simply not rational for the purposes of national security. Similarly, Maher's use of imagery from an oil spill does not acknowledge that it is oil companies, not religious groups, that have been responsible for spilling petroleum into the ocean. The images of violence included in the last segment of *Religulous* were in fact committed primarily by power-seeking nation-states and profit-seeking corporations. But coupled with Maher's apocalyptic narration, in which he suggests that religious beliefs threaten to bring about the end of the world, the images promote a fearful attitude toward religion.

My intention here is not to defend religion as "rational"—indeed, I find some religious beliefs and practices either positively or negatively irrational—or to defend violence motivated by religion. Rather, my point is that the destruction depicted in the film misleadingly suggests that religion is the primary source of irrational violence—a notion prevalent in the secular cultural imaginary. In turn, this bias has the unfortunate consequence of distracting us from the real source of so much irrational violence committed by states and corporations.

Critical questioning of the rhetoric of "rationality" resonates in the thought and works of acclaimed Minamata writer Ishimure Michiko. Ishimure critiques what she takes to be the essential telos of so-called rational thought: the primacy of accruing profits by any means necessary, coupled with the eschewing of responsibility for damage caused by that pursuit of profit.[12] As Ishimure conceives of it, "rationality" is a mode of thought and action that elevates individual (and corporate) accrual of wealth and power without respect to harm to other individuals, communities, or the natural environment. In doing so, it reduces humans, animals, and nature to commodities, or means for making commodities, within a market economy.

Ishimure's critique of "rationality" raises concerns justified by events such as the September 2019 acquittal of the three CEO defendants of TEPCO by the Tokyo district judge overseeing the Fukushima nuclear accident case. No one was held legally accountable in the criminal trial for the meltdown of the Fukushima Daiichi nuclear power plant, despite the forewarning from the engineers about the plant's need for a higher wall to protect the facility from a tsunami. TEPCO's negligence left the plant vulnerable, leading to an unprecedented scale of destruction of lives, environment, community, livelihoods, and indeed the entire future of the region stricken by radiation. Yet the court failed to assign legal responsibility, even though the plaintiffs offered evidence that proved the cause of the meltdown was not merely a natural force but the lack of appropriate safety measures. The largest nuclear accident in our history occurred as a result of prizing profit over the protection of lives. In this way, structural violence is exerted through corporate negligence motivated by profit. The criminal nature of such corporate violence, like so much state violence, too often fails to be recognized as such, as if pursuing profit at the expense of lives were rational.

At the same time, I acknowledge that religious beliefs can lead to violence as well—for example, 1995's Aum Shinrikyō attacks with sarin gas on the Tokyo subway, the Oklahoma City Bombing that same year, and the September 11, 2001, attacks on the United States, to name a few. But again, these facts do not cancel out violence committed by nation-states and corporations, or render their violence less significant. Then, one may wonder fundamental differences of those entities—religiously motivated groups, nation-states, and corporations—that brought forth destructions. This question leads to another of what constitutes the category of "religion," or a concept of religion that sets it aside from the categories of politics, economics, and so on. Examining Ishimure Michiko's life and literary works as a response to these questions will not only illustrate violence caused by states and corporations but also highlight the religious sensibility that enabled her to see violence done to the precarious population who were marginalized.

In this and the following chapter, thus, I wish to focus on the trajectory of Ishimure Michiko's life and literary works, examining the religious dimensions of Ishimure's thought as they are expressed in her descriptions of Minamata sufferers. Such religious dimensions foster a world otherwise, an enspirited world rooted in the modern world. We will find that Ishimure's religious sensibility was formed during a childhood spent amid vulnerable others—humans, nonhumans, and other-than-humans in positions of precarity. As we will recall, precarity, by Judith Butlers' thinking, names a "politically induced condition"[13] that applies to beings who are overlooked, dismissed, or denied sympathy, making them vulnerable to state and corporate (as well as religious) violence. By rendering the vulnerable visible, Ishimure illuminates the conditions by which modern institutions sustain themselves at the expense of those it renders precarious.

By giving voice to the precarious, otherwise remained invisible, Ishimure's writings endow them with a power—a "fragile" power. This power—however fragile it is in this world—enables us to recognize the precarity, which urges us to realize and confront the flaws of the modern system. The power that derives from the precarity can be dangerous to those who maintain the status quo, supported by the precarity, for it can undermine social stability by challenging the modern institution of the nation-state framework. In order to better understand Ishimure's unique prose style that has afforded her distinction and renown as a writer, this chapter delves into Ishimure's life and her emergence as a writer, followed by chapter 6 focusing on an analysis of her work, so as to better convey her vision of a world otherwise.

The overarching question of this chapter returns us to the one, raised by Butler, that confronted us in chapter 1: "What are the cultural barriers against which we struggle when we attempt to name, and so to bring under the rubric of the 'human,'" those whose lives have been rendered precarious.[14] What blinds us to the suffering of others and the conditions that give rise to this plight is the frame through which we see and understand the world. Lives are seen or go unseen, are recognized or go unrecognized according to frames that "allocate recognition differentially,"[15] creating cultural barriers that create conditions of precarity.

The vision of a world otherwise—one that would afford recognition of the vulnerable—requires not only an ontological shift of the sort discussed in chapter 4 but also an epistemological shift. We are conditioned by cultural norms to blind ourselves to the precariousness of those who the social system deems insignificant and irrelevant. So how can we come to discern those made vulnerable by the system of precarity? In the next two chapters, I argue that Ishimure's *oeuvre* offers a breakthrough in the epistemological impasse, serving as a literary tool to broaden our horizon for envisioning a world otherwise. The power of fragility embodied in Ishimure's depiction of the vulnerable opens up a frame for seeing those who are otherwise invisible.

THE EARLY LIFE OF ISHIMURE MICHIKO

Although Ishimure Michiko is known as a local Minamata writer, she was actually born in (present-day) Amakusa City on Amakusa Islands, across the Shiranui Sea from Minamata. She spent just the first three months of her life there. (In order to avoid confusion, in the following account of the first half of Ishimure's early life, prior to establishing herself as a writer, I shall refer to her as Michiko.) Michiko was born on March 11, 1927, the first daughter of Shiraishi Kametarō and Haruno.[16] Her parents met when Kametarō was working for Yoshida Matsutarō, Michiko's maternal grandfather. Matsutarō was a mason serving as a chief of a unit of construction workers. Matsutarō, along with his daughter Haruno and son-in-law Kametarō, had already moved to Minamata from Amakusa prior to Michiko's birth, but they moved back to Amakusa temporarily to complete a construction project already underway. It was for this reason that Michiko was born in Amakusa. After the completion of the construction project, the family, now with the newborn Michiko, returned to Minamata.

Matsutarō's business thrived in Minamata. The city was expanding, its population increasing with the growth of the Chisso Corporation. When Michiko was three, Matsutarō built a house large enough to accommodate Matsutarō's entire family and all his workers under its roof. It was located in a newly developing area of Minamata called Sakae-machi—a town in which many Chisso employees resided. With Minamata's transformation from a small fishing village into an industrialized city, the streets grew busier and livelier each day. Within the neighborhood was an entertainment district where prostitutes would come and go.[17]

Michiko was drawn to the women of this district; she found them beautiful and yet sad, for reasons she could not at the time comprehend. One day, she learned that one of the women had been stabbed to death by a teenaged boy from a well-off family in Minamata. Her heart ached as she considered the murder of this young woman. Adding to her emotional turmoil was the fact that she was friends with the perpetrator's younger brother. Shortly after this crime took place, Matsutarō's business was on the decline and Michiko's family moved out of the area. As a result, she knew little of the consequences of the murder case, learning only that her friend was being bullied on account of his brother's crime. Michiko was thus exposed at an early age both to the bright lights and dark shadows of Minamata—the upbeat atmosphere of an economically thriving city, accompanied by the depressing realities of those whose exploitation in brothels rendered their lives precarious.

The good times for Michiko's family did not last long. When Michiko was in the second grade, Matsutarō's business finally went bankrupt. Separated from her grandfather, Michiko's parents and her maternal grandmother (Matsutarō's wife) Moka moved to the northern part of the city, close to the sea, commonly called *tonton mura*, where her father built a hut on his own. *Tonton mura* is a derogatory epithet, indicating the residential area where people would raise pigs (*ton*) for a living—an occupation that was looked down upon.[18] Although this move required the family to adopt a frugal and restricted way of living, Michiko's life was enriched by proximity to the sea; spending time on the beach nurtured her mind, her closeness to nature a source of joy and wonder. In addition, looking after her grandmother, Moka, who was blind and suffered from mental illness, afforded Michiko the invaluable opportunity to learn from the older woman's wisdom.

Growing up in a poverty-stricken household, Michiko contemplated a future as a worker in a cotton spinning mill (a job that her mother had once undertaken), but the teachers at her school took notice of Michiko's intelligence and encouraged her to receive the necessary education to become a schoolteacher. Thanks to support from her family and teachers, she was able to enroll in a Minamata *jitsumu gakkō*, the equivalent of a present-day high school. At that time, Japan was deep into its war with China, and the Pacific War would soon break out with the attack on Pearl Harbor. As the war became more and more intense, male teachers at school were conscripted one after another to be sent to the battlefield. The resultant shortage of schoolteachers compelled schools to hire people like Michiko, then barely sixteen, to serve as substitute teachers.

Michiko's first assignment was at Taura elementary school. On her route to school, looking over the community from her train window, she observed deserted rice paddies and vegetable fields: the laborers who had worked them were now acting as soldiers. At school, students wore decrepit shoes that exposed their feet even on snowy days. Everything, and everyone, was exhausted. Nonetheless, teachers were instructed to promulgate belief in Japan's eventual victory. Michiko began to wonder why the war was repeatedly referred to as "sacred" in propaganda disseminated by the government. What were she and her fellow citizens fighting for? After myriad precious lives had been lost in and outside the empire, the war ended with Japan's emperor admitting defeat on August 15, 1945. Michiko was eighteen years old.

School resumed in the fall of 1945, and so did Michiko's commute. It was on the train that Michiko encountered a girl who appeared feeble and lost. Asking her name and age, Michiko discovered that the girl, though only three years her junior, was so small and fragile that she looked like a little girl. Learning that the girl had no place to go, Michiko felt compelled to bring her home.[19] Their life together lasted for about fifty days, after which Michiko's family sent the girl back to Kakogawa, in Hyogo prefecture, which she claimed was her home.[20] Later, at the age of nineteen, Michiko would write a short piece about this girl, entitled "*Tadeko no ki*," or "The Record of Tadeko," which would become her first composition.

In biographical and autobiographical accounts of Michiko, descriptions of her postwar years are sparse and vague. We do know, however, that she attempted to take her life a few times after the end of the war. The first attempt was immediately after the war; she ingested arsenic that she had taken from her school's science lab. Fortunately, she regurgitated the poison, which saved her life. Another unsuccessful attempt came on July 20, 1947, only four months after her marriage to Ishimure Hiroshi,[21] a junior high school teacher.[22] Later, after a third suicide attempt, she resigned from her work as a school teacher.[23] Much later, responding to the question of why she had tried to take her own life, Michiko replied, "I wanted to die. Nihilistic feelings always occupied my mind since I was little . . . partly because I disliked this world (*konoyo*). I still do."[24] Even when she was little, she felt that she did not belong to this world—a feeling that grew into her yearning for a world otherwise.

In the year following their marriage, Michiko and Hiroshi had their only child, a son they named Michio. While raising Michio, Michiko returned to writing, composing mainly poems, which she began submitting to local newspapers and journals. By 1956, she had become a member of a local poetry group, *Nanpū*. Around the same time, the poetry journal *Tanka kenkyū* awarded her their "New Writer of The Year" prize, recognizing Michiko as a promising young writer. Minamata's literary circle also began to acknowledge her work. Established writer and activist Tanigawa Gan invited Michiko to join his writers' group, *Sākuru mura,* suggesting that she submit her work to the group's quarterly journal of the same name. The journal *Sākuru mura* circulated throughout Kyushu Island with the objective of bringing together in its pages what was rendered marginal under the modern system, with its divisions of center and periphery, intellectuals and commoners, women and men, humans and nature. Approximately 200 coal miners, teachers, artisans, and housewives subscribed to the journal, which was published from 1958 to 2006. Inspired by some members of this group, Michiko joined the Communist Party in 1959, only to abandon it the next year, following Tanigawa Gan's departure.[25] Though Ishimure offers no comments on her short-lived affiliation with communism, it is likely she was looking for a way to address and redress the injustices she observed around her, but not in the political party.

In the meantime, Tanigawa's work had opened Michiko's eyes; she found his use of language irresistible. Visiting Fukuoka, 120 miles from her house in Minamata, for the Sākuru mura meetings, also inspired Michiko to write about the lives of coal miners, as one of Japan's largest coal mines, Chikuhō, was located in Fukuoka Prefecture. In the late nineteenth century and into the first half of the twentieth, a number of women and men worked in coal mines, despite the dangers and harshness of the job.[26] The demand for coal was high, but the working conditions were far from safe and satisfactory. By the time Michiko visited Chikuhō, the coal-mining industry in the area was suffering from the shift to oil; many mines had either been shut down or were on the brink of closing. Later, linking Minamata people's struggle to this experience of having witnessed the large yet empty facilities for mining and the disintegrating lives of the miners and their families, Michiko wrote, "When I went to the coal mine (in Chikuhō), it made sense why everyone went there to work. I learned later that Minamata sufferers, such as Kawamoto Teruo and Tanoue Yoshiharu, had all gone there at some point in their lives, since they could not continue fishing in Minamata and no other jobs were available to them there."[27] Though Chikuhō was only barely open, some still migrated from Minamata to look for a better life. By 1976, all the mines in the Chikuhō region had ceased operation completely.

Michiko began dedicating more of her time to writing. The more she devoted herself to literature, however, the more frustrated she grew with being a *shufu*, or stay-at-home wife. Not earning any income, she had to sell her belongings to pay for the train fare to attend Sākuru mura meetings in Fukuoka. She became more conscious of the conflict between her desire to meet society's expectations for a shufu—cooking, housekeeping, and childrearing—and to realize her aspirations as a writer. Her awareness of this inner struggle eventually distanced her from the ideals expressed in Tanigawa's works and from discussions in the group's meetings. She could no longer relate to the predominantly male members' interests and concerns. Feeling that she did not belong added a further sorrow to her struggle, but this strife would also lead to her finding a way to translate her own voice and perspective into writing.

Depleted by her duties and her disappointment, Michiko was unable to resist her suicidal impulses. At one point, she wrote in her journal that she would like to end her life with poison, while on another occasion she prepared a will, asking Hiroshi to find a better mother for their son, Michio.[28] What anchored Michiko to this world was a rather coincidental encounter with Minamata sufferers that occurred when she brought an ailing Michio to the hospital. Michio was diagnosed with tuberculosis and was soon hospitalized in Minamata City Hospital. It was there that Michiko came upon the sufferers, who were being treated for kibyō (strange disease). Witnessing their excruciating pain—both physical and emotional—compelled Michiko to write about the sufferers. Her essay, entitled *Kibyō*, appeared in *Sākuru mura* in January 1960. This work eventually served as a basis for her magnum opus, *Kugai jōdo: Waga Minamata no ki,* or *Paradise in the Sea of Sorrow: Our Minamata Disease.*

THE CITIZENS' MOVEMENT AND ISHIMURE MICHIKO'S RISE AS A WRITER

Ishimure Michiko—henceforth referred to as Ishimure—continued to work on the theme of kibyō, as evident in her next piece, "Sora to umi no aida de" (Between the sky and the sea). "Sora to umi" was written for a literary journal, *Kumamoto fudoki,* through which she met Watanabe Kyōji, who would become her lifelong friend. Watanabe immediately recognized Ishimure's gift and volunteered to be her editor; he eventually became her avid supporter as a coworker and caretaker. He believed that Ishimure's unique ability was to be able to relate to the suffering of the marginalized, those who were not mourned by society at large—from women in brothels to her own grandmother, children going barefoot in winter, a war orphan, coalminers and Minamata sufferers and their families.

Ishimure continued to visit Minamata sufferers in the hospital long after Michio had been discharged. One of her biographers, Yonemoto Kōji, describes the egregious discrimination against Minamata sufferers at the time: "When Minamata sufferers handed money to a store clerk, the clerk would not touch the money, as if touching it transmitted their disease. Then, the clerk would throw the received coins into boiling water for disinfection. When the sufferers walked by residences, those living there would often sprinkle disinfectant where the sufferers had stepped."[29] While many citizens mistreated the sufferers, ignoring or abusing them, Ishimure *saw* them, and sought to tell their stories in her literature.

In 1968, the Ministry of Welfare finally admitted that Minamata disease was not a sporadically occurring local disease or fishers' disease, but a *kōgaibyō*, an illness induced by environmental pollution. Since Chisso refused to negotiate directly with the sufferers, the Ministry of Welfare appointed a third party to negotiate the case. The involvement of a third party, however, provoked a further division among the sufferers, who subsequently broke into two factions. Eighty-nine sufferers from sixty-four households, called *ichinin-ha* (the arbitration group), chose to entrust negotiations to a third party, while forty-five sufferers from twenty-nine households were determined to pursue the case in court; they were called *jishu kōshō-ha,* or the direct negotiation group (later *soshō-ha*, or the trial group).[30] At first, the majority of Minamata citizens were far from being supportive of the sufferers because they believed that the sufferers were destroying Chisso, the city's economic foundation. Ishimure records their responses: "Are you going to bankrupt the company [Chisso]? If the company goes down, all of Minamata will sink with it. Which is more important—the lives of 45,000 Minamata citizens or the lives of a hundred or so Minamata sufferers?"[31] Writing of the derogations and accusations directed at the sufferers, Ishimure realized that the sufferers were killed twice: once by Chisso and again by their fellow citizens.

Ishimure's conversations with Minamata sufferers formed the basis of several novellas, which began to appear in *Sākuru mura* in 1960 and in *Kumamoto fudoki* from 1965 to 1966. A semi-fictional account of these compiled testimonies of the sufferers became Ishimure's 1969 book *Kugai jōdo: Waga Minamata no ki*.[32] The title, *Kugai jōdo,* was suggested by Ueno Eishin, a writer who presented Ishimure's manuscript to a prospective publisher. "Ueno-san proposed *Kugai* (the suffering world)," Ishimure recalled fondly, while Hiroshi asked how she "would like *jōdo* (Pure Land, a Buddhist term) following *kugai*. I liked those words together. It took less than three minutes to decide the title of the book."[33]

On April 17, 1969, the year *Kugai jōdo* was published, two men staged a sit-in demonstration in front of Chisso's Minamata factory. They were Watanabe Kyōji and Koyama Kazuo. Watanabe, as noted above, was Ishimure's lifelong editor and friend; Koyama was assisted in the operations of the English school run by Watanabe at the time. In the two days leading up to the demonstration, Watanabe distributed flyers in Kumamoto city, the capital of the prefecture, calling for people to join them at the demonstration in Minamata. Aside from Watanabe and Koyama, however, only three men participated in the demonstration: Handa Takashi, an employee of NHK, the national broadcasting station; Hisano Keisuke, a journalist from Kumamoto's local newspaper, *Kumamoto Nichinichi Shimbun*; and Ishimure's son, Michio. As Ishimure observed, although the demonstration attracted only a few attendees, it marked the beginning of a citizens' movement, in which individual citizens who had not contracted Minamata disease raised their voices against Chisso's injustice to the sufferers.

Despite the poor attendance, the demonstration had an impact on people in Kumamoto, who formed a group, *Minamatabyō o kokuhatsu suru kai* (the Association to Indict [Those Responsible for] Minamata disease, hereafter, Kokuhatsu suru kai) comprising thirty members only three days after the sit-in. Ishimure was one of them.[34] Kokuhatsu suru kai then filed a lawsuit against Chisso for compensation to the tune of 640 million Japanese yen. Honda Keikichi, one of the leading figures of Kokuhatsu suru kai, was uncomfortable with the legal language, which he found to be insufficient to the sense of loss and frustration on the part of the plaintiff. He therefore tried to use language that expressed their feelings more directly and reflected their experiences more accurately, even though such language was regarded as unsuitable in court. "The lawyers," he said, "advised us to leave behind our personal resentment in court, but, for us, this lawsuit was a vendetta [*adauchi*]—fighting for the dead and the harmed. We were in court for the righteousness of our cause [*gi ni yotte sukedachi itasu*]."[35]

Abandoning personal grievances defeated the purpose of the entire lawsuit in the eyes of the sufferers. The conventional language of the court seeks to exclude emotions; supposedly, objective language is intended to remove raw emotion from proceedings. But in his deliberation, Honda included words like *vendetta* and *righteousness* (*gi*)—words recalling a premodern and non-Western moral code. In doing so, he seeks to move beyond the conventions that define the foundation of the modern legal system.

Honda's choice of language—one that bypasses the norms of the legal system in its foregrounding of emotions—is observed in Ishimure's work as well. Ishimure adopts the Minamata dialect when the sufferers talk about their plight. The language in her work does not strictly reflect the Minamata dialect; rather, Ishimure amalgamates the local dialect with standard Japanese in creating her own "Michiko dialect" legible to general readers. Preserving the local dialect was crucial for Ishimure, who wished to convey the sufferers' raw emotions and the gravity of the sufferers' plight. But the use of a local dialect also functionally resists standard language, which, is more than merely a medium of communication, is also a mechanism for reproducing social order, delegitimating uses of language that deviate from it. It is for this reason that local dialects are often devalued, in both oral communication and in literature, as the mark of the uneducated or unsophisticated. Ishimure's strategic use of local language, like Honda's, marks a refusal to be incorporated within the social order that represses those on whose behalf she speaks.

Ishimure continued to submit her writings to journals, one of which was Kokuhatsu suru kai's newsletter *Kokuhatsu.* For the article in *Kokuhatsu,* Ishimure reported on Kamimura Tomoko, who at the time was thirteen years old but whose mobility and speech had been impaired because of her exposure to mercury in utero. Her parents, the plaintiffs in the trial, brought Tomoko with them to the court. When Tomoko cried out in the middle of the trial, the judge ordered her father to leave the room with Tomoko because her cry disrupted the proceedings. Instead of listening to the cry of one of the most innocent victims of the case, the judge prioritized order in the court over the voice of the vulnerable. The outcry of the sufferer—whose condition Ishimure describes as "ikitoru manma shinda ningen" (being killed but but also kept alive)—in the midst of a trial seeking to assign responsibility for suffering, awakened Ishimure to the inadequacy of the legal system, its language, and its order.[36]

Ishimure speculated that the judge may have feared that Tomoko's powerful presence would nullify his authority, which was sustained by the modern system. After all, who would be a better witness to the case than Tomoko? Unlike the judge, to Ishimure's ears, Tomoko's cry sounded as "a song, a weeping, or a bubble. That was the voice of a 'person who is killed but also kept alive'"[37] When Ishimure's works appeared in *Kokuhatsu,* Watanabe admiringly confessed, they influenced the group's aptitude and writings: "Ishimure Michiko's thoughts and ideals [*rinen*] had become those of *Kokuhatsu.*"[38]

In the meantime, the arbitration group, which had chosen to work with the third party appointed by the national government, was also working with *Minamatabyō hoshō shori iinkai*, the Minamata Disease Compensation Committee (hereafter the Committee). The group expected the compensation to be around three million yen, comparable to the amount paid to the bereaved families of other industrial accidents at the time. However, the Committee offered the much lower amount of 100,000 yen (approximately 914.41 US dollars in today's currency) for an adult, 30,000 yen for a child, and 300,000 yen for families of the bereaved.[39] In addition to the insultingly small amount of the offer, the arbitration group was further humiliated when it discovered that the group would have to consent to the proviso that Chisso would not be responsible for any additional payments following the settlement.

Fearing that the demeaning settlement would set an unfavorable example, the direct negotiation group and the Kokuhatsu suru kai came forward to support the arbitration group. In the face of the contemptuous treatment of the sufferers, Watanabe suggested that Kokuhatsu suru kai should stand in solidarity with them by occupying the meeting room assigned for the Committee's use. Ishimure joined these efforts, distributing flyers in front of the building where the Committee's meetings were held. As a result of this protest, thirteen members of Kokuhatsu suru kai were arrested. But their action garnered national attention, leading to payouts from eight to twenty times more than the original offer. By the conclusion of the settlement, Kokuhatsu suru kai was nationally known, winning supporters in major cities including Kyoto, Osaka, Nagoya, and Fukuoka.

In July 1970, attorney Gotō Takanori proposed *hitokabu undō* or the one-share movement. Gotō had been asked to undertake the Minamata case in 1968. Although circumstances prevented him from undertaking the case at the time, two years later, he was asked once again, via a different client. This time, he decided to take the case. Gotō himself thought that the court did not adequately represent the plaintiffs' wish, which was to restore the sufferers' dignity. As the first step toward this restoration of dignity, the plaintiffs sought firsthand interaction with Chisso's president.[40] In the past, the dismissal of their request to meet the president had provoked the sufferers to act out, resulting in chaos—labeled as a "riot"—and leading to arrests.[41] To avoid falling into the same trap, Gotō conceived a plan. Believing that a shareholders' meeting would provide an occasion for the sufferers to confront the company's executives,[42] Gotō purchased 10,000 shares of Chisso for 350,000 yen. At a Tokyo branch meeting of Kokuhatsu suru kai, his proposal that others also purchase shares, thereby allowing them to attend the shareholders' meeting, was unanimously supported.[43] In the end, members of Kokuhatsu suru kai's Tokyo, Osaka, Fukuoka, and Kumamoto branches acquired 50,000 shares altogether, with Minamata sufferers and Kumamoto members owning 13,300 shares.[44]

Chisso's autumn shareholders' meeting was to be held at Osaka's Kōsei Nenkin Hall on November 28, 1970. Thanks to the researches of Komatsubara Orika, a criminologist focusing on restorative justice, we can read Gotō's handwritten memo in which he expresses the overwhelming pressure of the daunting battle before him, which he felt was like "fighting against nuclear arms with bare hands."[45] To attend this meeting, the sufferers extemporaneously came up with the idea of donning white robes and white gloves, burial garment that became common attire for pilgrims of the Edo period, when travel entailed risking one's life. Nothing could have been more appropriate than the white outfit for the travelers from Minamata to Osaka, who were "being killed twice" once by methylmercury from Chisso and then by discrimination in their communities.[46] Over their white robes, they wore sashes emblazoned with the words, *Minamatabyō kanja junreidan* (Minamata disease sufferers on a pilgrimage). Inspired by a city staff member who had come with a black flag to the funeral of Ishimure's father, Kametarō,

Ishimure suggested that the sufferers carry a black flag with the word *on* (grievance) appearing in white letters.

On the day of the meeting, the sufferers and supporters gathered in Osaka in their white robes and sashes, carrying their black flag.[47] Seated on the second floor of the meeting room, they chanted "*Goeika*," a Buddhist pilgrim song, which they had rehearsed for that day, despite speech and sight impairments deriving from the disease. When the meeting began, the sufferers and Kokuhatsu suru kai members could not resist rushing the stage where Chisso executives were seated. Facing them up close and in person for the first time, the sufferers spontaneously cried out, "Drink! Drink mercury!"[48]

Among these sufferers was Hamamoto Fumiyo, who, though known to be quiet and reserved, on this day held up her parents' mortuary tablets to then-president Egashira Yutaka.[49] "These are my parents! . . . Do you understand how I feel . . . having lost my parents to mercury poisoning?" "I am Hamamoto, Hamamoto from Dezuki! Do you understand my feelings? My heart? Do you understand?"[50] But Egashira completely ignored the presence of Fumiyo and the other sufferers. Gotō's revised agenda, proposing to address the sufferers' plight, was also dismissed before he could finish reading it aloud; the meeting was brought to a close after only four minutes. Enraged, the sufferers yelled at Egashira, demanding that he take to his knees to apologize.[51] The turmoil continued until Ishimure grabbed a microphone and addressed the sufferers, concluding: "Let's go home."[52]

The actual meeting was far from the human interaction that the sufferers had anticipated, yet the impact of what was to be called the "one-share movement" was immense. The companies' shares had previously been sold on the market in units of 500 or 1,000. To make the shares affordable to as many supporters as possible, Gotō had purchased them in units and broken them up into single shares. Subsequent to this meeting, however, Chisso decided to charge a commission for dividing the shares. In 1981, the commercial law was also changed, requiring a shareholder to own more than 50,000 yen of shares in order to attend the meeting.[53]

The movement, as powerful as it was, did not avoid criticism. Some were skeptical that attending the shareholders' meeting would contribute to any practical change in favor of the sufferers. Others argued that by buying Chisso's shares, the sufferers and supporters would become a part of Chisso. One of these critics was Yamamoto Shigeo, the lead counsel for the plaintiff, who expressed his concern that joining such a movement might cause the judge to look upon them unfavorably—a concern that provoked a sense of guilt among the sufferers. Urging the sufferers not to appear as troublemakers, Yamamoto said, "Do you think that the spirits in heaven (*ten no rei*) would want you to complain to Chisso's executives for not mourning over you? Given the irremediable losses you have suffered, I think that the spirits in heaven want us to build a stable life for ourselves by obtaining as much compensation as possible."[54] Yamamoto thus sounds a note of sympathy, even as he discourages his vulnerable clients from pursuing the firsthand interactions that they believed would bring them relief.

Ishimure supported the one-share movement, explained the significance of the shareholder meeting. She believed that joining the movement was a healing process for the sufferers, whose dignity had been relentlessly eroded by pains both from the disease and the legal procedure. Facing the responsible party and expressing their emotions (which the court had forbidden) were necessary for them in order to come to terms with the assault to their dignity. What they had lost was not only their loved ones and their own health but also their livelihoods, their community, and their relations to their environment. Admonishing sufferers not to be emotional, not to cry out, and not to be troublemakers was, to Ishimure, another way of dismissing the sufferers' plight—or worse, of discounting the harm done to them. Ishimure did not deny the meaning of the lawsuit but knew what the sufferers wanted the most was to meet the Chisso executives. The sufferers' emotions had been neglected and delegitimized in court, and the one-share movement, their only remaining "official" means for meeting Chisso executives, had been made illegal.

Having experienced the disappointment of corporate regulations and commercial laws changing to the benefit of those in power while failing to accommodate their own needs, the Minamata sufferers and their supporters had to find yet another means by which to pursue their demands. On December 8, 1971, a year after the Minamata sufferers' meeting with Egashira, approximately 200 members of both Kokuhatsu suru kai and the direct negotiation group, led by Kawamoto Teruo, laid siege to the president's office at Chisso headquarters in Tokyo. This time, they managed to converse in person with Chisso's president, Shimada Ken'ichi. Kawamoto petitioned Chisso to pay 30 million yen to each sufferer, irrespective of the duration of suffering or severity of symptoms. Upon Shimada's repeated refusal to meet this demand, Kawamoto finally implored Shimada literally to seal the petition with his own blood: "Cut your finger, now!" Shimada remained steadfast in his refusal. Ishimure was in the room and witnessed the negotiation. Later, she wrote about the frustration that characterized this period during which the appeal was not heard by Chisso at all. Instead, the sufferers' claim was described by critics as a way to extort more money by resorting to what they characterized as a physical threat. But having been treated as utterly insignificant, Kawamoto and others had simply asked for the word of Shimada himself, as a representative of Chisso, in a manner modeled after Japan's premodern custom of *keppan*, or seal of blood.

All said, the negotiations lasted for twenty months, during which time the supporters put up a tent in front of Chisso's headquarters in Tokyo, among the high rises. To report back to those who stayed behind in Minamata, the supporters in Tokyo issued a daily newsletter, *Nikkan Chisso*. The punning title exploits the homophonic duplicity of "Chisso," which can mean either "nitrogen" or "source of shame." The newsletter uses the Chinese characters for the latter—thus, the *Daily Source of Shame*. One of Ishimure's articles, appearing in issue no. 16, on January 27, 1972, of *Nikkan Chisso*, articulates the meaning of the sufferers' relentless demand for a face-to-face meeting with Chisso executives: "What is the meaning of pursuing direct negotiation at Chisso headquarters in Tokyo? It is quite simple. Those who were killed will not be able to rest in peace until they have been heard by their killers. . . . All of us are here in order to relay the voices of the dead. Facing the killers, the sufferers here feel anger—their own and that of the dead."[55]

In referring to the dead, Ishimure often uses the term *Minamata shimin*, "the citizens of Minamata." But in doing so, she renders the phrase with Chinese characters meaning "the dead citizens of Minamata." For the sufferers and supporters, the presence of the dead was palpable, a sentiment manifesting in their exploitation of linguistic double meanings of "Chisso" and "shimin." In their actions and in their words, the living sufferers were keenly aware that they fought for, and with, the dead.

During these months in Tokyo, joining the sufferers and supporters on the street, Ishimure gained invaluable perspective by sleeping on a bundle of newspapers as a pillow and gathering fallen leaves to cover herself against the cold on the city street. Recalling those days, she remarks, "The street [I slept on] was not soil but asphalt, which was much colder. But I treasured the experiences as I felt so human then." The journalist Yonemoto Kōji asked Ishimure why those experiences made her feel "human." Ishimure replied, "Because from the street, I had to look up to people walking by and the buildings towering overhead. . . . Chisso workers frowned upon us, and some even spat on us. It was difficult, but, at the same time, I felt closer to the sufferers who had been shoved down to such a lowly place." "The experience, comparable to being a *kanjin,* or beggar," continued Ishimure, "was good for me. I had always wished to be a beggar."[56] With this remark, Ishimure conveys a sense of the "human" that stands at a far remove from the person conceived as an autonomous and self-sufficient entity conditioned by modern legal, social, economic, and political systems. Rather, she conceives of the human as one who is with the dead, and who is helpless, asking for help, like a beggar—or like an actant in an assemblage.[57]

Although the trial, by its nature, focused on negotiating compensation monies, the sufferers knew that they were fighting for more than money. At the end of the lawsuit, Honda encapsulated the forty-three plaintiff's voices, declaring, "We do not need the money; give us back our parents. Give us back our bodies, healthy and sound. Give us back the Shiranui Sea. Undo the pollution."[58] Ishimure also records their outcries when Judge Saitō Jirō stated that "the agreement on a compensation has brought reconciliation." Hearing this, the sufferers began to exclaim, "I will buy your life! Let's have fun. I will buy your life with the compensation money!" "With that money, I will buy your arm. I will buy your leg. I will bring you to Minamata."[59] Their shouts revealed what they really wanted most: They wanted Chisso executives to feel their anger, sadness, and frustration—emotions that the court was unable to address. They wanted the executives to understand what it was like to lose their loved ones to agonizing deaths, to lose control over their bodies, to lose their livelihoods, to lose respect in the community, and to lose their dignity as human beings. That, and not merely money, was what they had demanded from the beginning. But of course, what the trial revealed was the cold fact that the legal system was in no way designed to address the sufferers' emotional demands nor to retrieve their lost humanity.

In March 1973, the Minamata district court gave a final verdict in favor of the plaintiff of the direct negotiation group, which was commonly referred to as the *daiichiji soshō,* or the first trial. Although the end of this trial hardly brought closure to the Minamata sufferers' plight, the publication of the *Kokuhatsu* newsletter discontinued after the August issue, and in its place a new publication, *Minamata*, arose. This was the year that Ishimure left her husband in Minamata in order to pursue her life as a writer in Kumamoto city.[60] She became involved in a new quarterly literary journal, *Kuragou*, which published fiction and essay dedicated to matters of social and environmental justice. Here Ishimure worked alongside the journal's founders, Watanabe and a writer named Matsuura Toyotoshi, who had been a prominent supporter of Kokuhatsu suru kai while running a coffee shop, *Karigari*, in Kumamoto city, where the members of Kokuhatsu suru kai often gathered. *Kuragou* produced forty-eight volumes before its discontinuation in 1992, marking the end of a long phase of legal and political struggle and anticipating the formation of Hongan no kai and its efforts to realize a world otherwise.

This chapter has traced Ishimure's life into her early seventies, as well as the struggles of Minamata sufferers. Before her passing on February 10, 2018, and despite her twenty-year struggle with Parkinson's disease, Ishimure continued to produce her literary work, including novels, a serial story in a newspaper, two Noh plays, interviews, and letters. Throughout her life, she was always attentive to the marginalized and vulnerable. As historian of Japanese thought Mizutamari Mayumi states, "Across her work, Minamata is described by Ishimure as a world of the dispossessed and of migrants from Amakusa, outside the world of Chisso and its employees."[61]

But Ishimure did not embrace an idealized premodern or rural vision of community, as she was keenly aware of the complex forms of discrimination that too often characterized such communities, as we saw in chapters 2 and

3. Nor did she merely describe a mythic world where spirits and deities play. As Watanabe insightfully reveals, Ishimure's world is conjured up when the marginalized, or those who find nowhere to belong, interact with and transform this present, modern world.[62] A world otherwise is not an independent and autonomous world, but rather one that appears in and interacts with this world. It is for this reason that those depicted in Ishimure's works are vulnerable—but powerful for that very reason. With a voice given by Ishimure, they serve a critical purpose, revealing possibilities for subverting the systems and structures that have rendered their lives precarious. They are treated as insignificant and irrelevant in this world, yet precisely because of their marginalized status, they indicate ways of realizing values different from those of market economy. With this in mind, chapter 6 will examine Ishimure's works, which reveal the space between this world and a world otherwise.

NOTES

1. *Religulous,* directed by Larry Charles. 2008.

2. Among the critiques made for the category and conception of "religion" in religious studies are, for example, Talal Asad in *Genealogies of Religion: Discipline and Reasons of Power in Christianity and Islam* (Baltimore, MD: Johns Hopkins University Press, 2013), Tomoko Masuzawa in *The Invention of World Religions, or, How European Universalism Was Preserved in the Language of Pluralism* (Chicago: University of Chicago Press, 2005), and Thomas A. Lewis, *Why Philosophy Matters for the Study of Religion & Vice Versa* (New York: Oxford University Press, 2015). For example, "For many, this focus on belief and faith derives at least in large part from the Protestant Reformation's emphasis on faith." Lewis, *Why Philosophy Matters,* 3.

3. Peter McGraw and Jowl Warner, "The Danish Cartoon Crisis of 2005 and 2006: 10 Things You Didn't Know About the Original Muhammad Controversy," *Huffington Post,* September 24, 2012 (updated December 6, 2017).

4. Saba Mahmood, "Religious Reason and Secular Affect: An Incommensurable Divide?" in *Is Critique Secular? Blasphemy, Injury, and Free Speech,* eds. by Talal Asad, Wendy Brown, Judith Butler, and Saba Mahmood (Berkeley, CA: University of California Press, 2009), 64–100.

5. Mahmood, "Religious Reason and Secular Affect," 76.

6. Mahmood, "Religious Reason and Secular Affect," 66, 69.

7. Mahmood, "Religious Reason and Secular Affect," 74.

8. Mahmood, "Religious Reason and Secular Affect," 73.

9. Mahmood, "Religious Reason and Secular Affect," 83.

10. William T. Cavanaugh analyzes this association of religion and violence, which was, he reveals, rooted in the Western colonization project. See William T. Cavanaugh, *The Myth of Religious Violence* (New York: Oxford University Press, 2009).

11. In comparison to the 1,032 tests done by the United States, North Korea has conducted six tests, India two, and Pakistan one.

12. "Ishimure Michiko san ni kiku" (Asking Ishimure Michiko), *Tamashii utsure* 41, 2010: 13.

13. Butler, *Frames of War*, 28.

14. Butler, *Precarious Life*, 46.

15. Butler, *Frames of War*, 6.

16. *Nihonjin wa nani o mezashite kitanoka Chi no kyojin tachi* (What did Japan aim at? Intellectual giants), vol. 6, *Kindai towa nanika, Tamashii no yukue, Sakka Ishimure Michiko* (What is modernity? The whereabouts of the spirit, the writer Ishimure Michiko), aired January 17, 2015 on NHK. According to this documentary, Michiko had an older brother who was believed to have died in the battle of Okinawa.

17. I use the term "prostitute" as opposed to the more current "sex worker" in order to maintain the sense of immorality associated with people in this line of work at the time.

18. Those who skinned cows and horses faced discrimination in Japan's feudal system, ranking below the four strata of samurai (warriors), farmers, artisans, and merchants. The name *tonton mura* derived either from the residents' occupation of raising pigs (*ton*) or from the onomatopoeia of the *ton ton* (bang, bang) sound caused by hammering down the skin after the livestock were flayed.

19. Ishimure, Michiko, *Yoshi no Nagisa: Ishimure Michiko jiden* (The beach of the common reed: The autobiography of Ishimure Michiko) (Tokyo: Fujiwara shoten, 2014), 227.

20. Ishimure, *Yoshi no Nagisa,* 231–32.

21. Hiroshi was Michiko's brother's friend. After their marriage was fixed, she learned that Hiroshi's father, uncle, and two of his brothers worked for Chisso.

22. Kurihara, Akira and Fujiwara, Tatsushi, "Keshō no oto o kiku" (Listen to the nonhuman and other-than human beings), *Gendai shisō* 46, no. 7 (2019): 73. No record is available of Michiko's second suicide attempt, but sociologist Kurihara Akira recalls that Ishimure once said that she was going into the woods to kill herself.

23. Yonemoto, Kōji, *Hyouden Ishimure Michiko: Nagisa ni tatsu hito* (Critical Biography of Ishimure Michiko: A Person Who Stands on the Beach) (Tokyo: Shinchōsha, 2017), 65–66.

24. Yonemoto, *Hyouden Ishimure Michiko,* 68.

25. Ishimure, *Yoshi no nagisa,* 317.

26. In 131 mines in the area, 148,300 were working as miners in 1948. The number of workers declined as the energy source shifted from coals to petroleum. Takahashi Shin'ichi and Wakabayashi Yoshikazu, "Tankou roudousha no idou to kyū santanchi no shakai hendou" (Social Change and Labor Mobility in the Coal Industry), Bukkyo daigaku *Shakaigaku kenkyūsho kiyou* 11 (1990), 48.

27. Yonemoto, *Hyouden Ishimure Michiko,* 90.

28. Yonemoto, *Hyouden Ishimure Michiko,* 67.

29. Yonemoto, *Hyouden Ishimure Michiko*, 100.

30. Yahagi, Tadashi, "Chisso shi 1970–75, I" (The History of Chisso 1970–75, I), *Urawa Ronsō* 33 (2004): 53.

31. Yonemoto, *Hyouden Ishimure Michiko*, 156.

32. Ishimure, Michiko, *Paradise in the Sea of Sorrow: Our Minamata Disease*, trans. Livia Monnet (Ann Arbor, MI: Center for Japanese Studies, University of Michigan, 2003).

33. Yonemoto, *Hyouden Ishimure Michiko,* 124. Thus, *Kugai jōdo* literally means the suffering world and pure land, but the English translation by Livia Monnet, *Paradise in the Sea of Sorrow* captured Minamata sufferers' experiences and their yearning for an alternative world.

34. Watanabe's involvement in the demonstration and in this newly founded group was a surprise to people who knew him, however, as by then he tended to distance himself from political activities. What urged him to take action was his encounter the work of Ishimure, who had been friends with him for four years. Yonemoto, *Houden Ishimure Michiko,* 149–153.

35. Yonemoto, *Hyouden Ishimure Michiko*, 156.

36. Yonemoto, *Hyouden Ishimure Michiko*, 159.

37. Yonemoto, *Hyouden Ishimure Michiko*, 159.

38. Yonemoto, *Hyouden Ishimure Michiko*, 157.

39. Yonemoto, *Hyouden Ishimure Michiko*, 159.

40. Gotō, Takanori, *Chinmoku to bakuhatsu: dokyumento "Minamatabyō jiken" 1873–1995* (Silence and Explosion: Document Minamata disease incident 1873–1995) (Tokyo: Shūeisha, 1995), 138–140.

41. Komatsubara, Orika, "'Higaisha no jōnen' kara 'higaisha no hyōgen' e: Minamatabyō 'hitokabu undō' (1970) ni okeru higaisha・kagaisha taiwa o kentou suru" (From 'victims' passions' to 'victims' expressions': Examination of the victims/victimizers dialogue on the Minamatabyō one-share movement [1970]), *Gendai seimei tetsugaku kenkyū* 8 (2019): 64. Also see Togashi Sadao, *Minamatabyō jiken to hou* (The Minamata disease incident and the law) (Fukuoka: Sekifūsha, 1995), 64.

42. Gotō thought of this idea while he was bathing. See Komatsubara, "'Higaisha no jōnen' kara 'higaisha no hyōgen' e," 68–69.

43. "Jinsei no okurimono: Hitokabu undo de Chisso no shakaiteki sekinin o tou" (A gift of life: Imputing Chisso's social responsibility through the one-share movement: An interview with Gotō Takanori), *Asahi Shimbun*, October 26, 2009.

44. "Kanja daihyō ni kabu watasu" (Giving the shares to the sufferers' representative), *Kumamoto nichinichi Shimbun,* October 31, 1970.

45. Komatsubara, "'Higaisha no jōnen' kara 'higaisha no hyōgen' e," 73. In fact, the "pilgrims" from Minamata stopped at Hiroshima to visit the Hiroshima Peace Museum.

46. Yonemoto, *Hyouden Ishimure Michiko,* 156.

47. According to Gotō, the day of the meeting, he wrapped his abdomen with newspaper and bandages (Iwataobi, used for the pregnant women), in case of the right wing's attack. Police officers were surrounding the building. Gotō, *Chinmoku to bakuhatsu,* 145–146.

48. Yonemoto, *Hyouden Ishimure Michiko,* 166.

49. Egashira's father-in-law was Navy admiral, Yamaya Tanin, and Egashira's granddaughter is Owada Masako, who later married Naruhito, the current emperor since 2019.

50. Tsuchimoto, "*Minamata—Kanjasan to sono sekai,*" cited in Komatsubara, "'Higaisha no jōnen' kara 'higaisha no hyōgen' e," 103.

51. Komatsubara, "'Higaisha no jōnen' kara 'higaisha no hyōgen' e," 59. Despite the chaos, Egashira reported to other shareholders that the meeting went smoothly. Later, Gotō filed a lawsuit to overturn the meeting's decisions due to the disorder at the meeting. His suit prevailed at all the court levels: local, regional, and supreme.

52. Komatsubara, "'Higaisha no jōnen' kara 'higaisha no hyōgen' e," 167–168.

53. This regulation was revised again in 2018.

54. Tsuchimoto, "Minamata, cited in Komatsubara, "'Higaisha no jōnen' kara 'higaisha no hyōgen' e," 80.

55. Ishimure, Michiko, "Saranaru shien o! Jishu kōshō no imi" (More support needed! The significance of the direct negotiation), *Nikkan Chisso* 16 (1972).

56. Yonemoto, *Hyouden Ishimure Michiko*, 220–221.

57. Bennett, *Vibrant Matter*, 8–10.

58. Yonemoto, *Hyouden Ishimure Michiko*, 172.

59. Yonemoto, *Hyouden Ishimure Michiko,* 173.

60. Her son Michio had already left for college in Nagoya.

61. Mizutamari, Mayumi, "Ishimure Michiko to 'rumin'" (Ishimure Michko and the Displaced) *Gendai shisō* 46, no. 7 (2018): 192.

62. Watanabe, Kyōji, *Mou hitotsu no konoyo: Ishimure Michiko no uchū* (A World Otherwise: Ishimure Michiko's cosmos) (Fukuoka: Gen shobō, 2013), 51.

Chapter 6

Genius Loci and the Discourse of Home

EARTH SPIRIT AND TOKYO SKY TREE

At 634 meters in height, the Tokyo Sky Tree telecommunications tower literally towers over metropolitan Tokyo. The building was completed in 2012 and was acknowledged by Guinness World Records as the world's tallest building that same year. Today, the Sky Tree is no longer the tallest structure in the world, but it remains the tallest communications tower.[1] The construction of the tower required advanced technology, sophisticated engineering, and intricate architectural methods, in order to endure earthquakes caused by the active fault lines that run beneath the Japanese archipelago. The chief client of this project was NHK, along with five other commercial television stations in Tokyo. Given the modern trappings of the project, one might, therefore, be surprised to learn that a religious ritual accompanied the inauguration of its construction in 2008. Representatives of the involved parties—the clients, construction company, and a group of architects—attended a Shinto ritual called *jichinsai* as part of the groundbreaking ceremony.

Jichinsai is a ritual intended to pacify the earth spirit, as is suggested by its other name, *toko shizume no matsuri* or "ritual to appease the ground." Descriptions of this ritual appear as far back the mythical and historical record *Nihon shoki* (720 CE) and the Shinto source, *Kogo shūi* (807 CE). To this day, the ritual is widely performed and observed in Japan as part of groundbreaking ceremonies for the construction of private homes and corporate buildings. This ritual is conventionally conducted in the Shinto style, with the presence of Shinto priests.[2] This was the case with the Tokyo Sky Tree's jichinsai, where a priest from the neighboring Ushijima Shinto shrine conducted the ritual. As part of the ritual, a construction site is enclosed with a rice-straw rope (*shimenawa*) to demarcate the sacred space from its profane surroundings. Within the roped-off space, a wooden altar is assembled on which saké, water, rice, salt, vegetables, and sometimes fish are displayed as offerings.

Looking up at the modern tower, one may wonder why secular companies in a supposedly secular society continue hosting religious rituals at the outset of construction, and why still today both Shinto and Buddhist rituals continue to be enacted as means for pacifying the *chirei*, or *genius loci*—the earth spirit, or spirit of a specific place. In a country where, in response to a 2018 survey, sixty-two percent of the population claimed that they did not believe in any particular religion,[3] jichinsai is still widely practiced.[4] The survival of this ritual suggests that people's belief in the earth spirit, which originated in folkloric and animistic traditions, so widely prevailed that Shinto and Buddhism adopted it, integrating corresponding rituals into their practices. Nonetheless, the ritual is hardly registered as a "religious" activity, which explains the 2018 survey. The widespread occurrence of jichinsai on the one hand, and over sixty percent of the population claiming to hold no religious beliefs on the other lead us to ask what this ritual might tell us about the standing of religion in Japan. In examining Ishimure Michiko's distinctive writing style, this chapter argues that the persistence of these religious beliefs and rituals demonstrates an awareness of and respect for other-than-humans, in particular, earth spirits. This religious sensibility also forms the basis of Ishimure's contribution to environmental ethics.

ISHIMURE'S MYTHOPOETIC WRITING

Ishimure, who died in 2018 at the age of ninety from acute exacerbation of the Parkinson's disease, wrote prolifically into the 1990s. In 1994, Ishimure, as a founding member of Hongan no kai, a collective comprising Minamata sufferers' and supporters, remained active in the group, even as her health deteriorated due to the Parkinson's disease in the late 1990s. In 1982, she published *Ayatori no ki* (The account of cat's cradle), a semiautobiographical novel in which a little girl, Micchin, interacts with people such as Iwadon, a crematorium worker; Hiromu Niiyan, a tall orphan; and Secchan, a beggar who always has a puppy clutched in her arms. Here as elsewhere, Ishimure focuses on socially marginalized characters and their interactions with other-than-humans. *Oen yugyō* (Oen's pilgrimage), published in 1984, tells the story of a mentally disturbed female beggar who maintains a special relationship with a spirit—she calls it Nyama—that resides in her bosom. Ishimure's collection of poems about Minamata sufferers, *Umi to sora no aida ni* (Between the sky and the sea), appeared in 1989. Eight years later, she published *Tenko* (Lake of Heaven), in which a young man from Tokyo rediscovers himself in his grandfather's home village, which is not submerged in the bottom of water, with the help of local shamans.

Ishimure's 1999 novel, *Anima no tori* (The bird of anima), originally published as *Haru no shiro* in 1998, was based on the historical event *Shimabara no ran*, known as the Shimabara-Amakusa Rebellion (1637–1638), a protest against the officer of the local domain's oppressive politics and excessive taxation. Eventually, after losing many lives, the rebellion was suppressed by the Tokugawa shogunate. Ishimure offers an imaginative recounting of the event, portraying not the heroic warriors, but on common people living on the Amakusa Islands. Ishimure, who was born on the main island of Amakusa, describes the religious culture there—an amalgamation of Christianity, True Pure Land Buddhism, and local folk beliefs. In the meantime, *Tsubaki no umi no ki* (Story of the Sea of Camellias, 1976) and *Kugai jōdo* (Paradise in the sea of sorrow, 1969) were translated into English by Livia Monnet and published in 1983 and 1990, respectively. These two semi-fictional accounts, like others that will be treated below, detail the lives of Minamata sufferers, whose spiritual sensibilities mingle Buddhist beliefs and local fishers' folk religion. As this abbreviated selection of her works suggests, Ishimure foregrounds characters whose lives are precarious.

Throughout her career as a writer who was concerned with environmental degradations, Ishimure was often compared to conservationist and biologist Rachel Carson, author of the 1962 classic of environmentalist writing, *Silent Spring*.[5] Although they focused on different causes of environmental degradation—Carson wrote on chemical pesticides and Ishimure on methylmercury—both authors elevated environmental consciousness in and beyond their respective societies. Their writings differ in other respects, however; not only their subjects but their approaches, or prose styles, are markedly different. Carson's prose is the lucid, journalistic, and factual writing of a scientist—a marine biologist. Ishimure's oeuvre, by contrast, mingles fact and fantasy, having been described as "mythopoetic,"[6] and rife with "lyrical . . . rhythmic [and] poetic" prose.[7] Ishimure's style—whether writing fiction, semi-fiction, or nonfiction—was shaped by those whom she wrote about: people whose precariousness too often goes unrecognized, and whose deaths go ungrieved. For Ishimure, writing about people relegated to the margins of society allowed her to discover the richness of their worlds. In portraying these people, Ishimure eschews strict realism, evolving a mythopoetic mode that conjures the spirits and the sense of awe before the natural environment that characterizes their world.

Bruce Allen, who translated Ishimure's book *Tenko* into the English *Lake of Heaven*, recounts the American poet and environmental activist Gary

Snyder's description of Ishimure's work. Underscoring the "mythopoetic" quality of the writing, Snyder describes Ishimure's novels as having a "Noh flavor" that presents "much of the ancient lore of Japan and the lore of the spirit world."[8] Noh plays, as we will discuss below, take place in the overlapping space of two dimensions of existence—the profane world of everyday life and the world of spirits. Thus, in the terms, I have set out in this book, what Snyder refers to as the "Noh flavor" has to do with Ishimure's evocation of the multiple dimensions of her characters' lived realities. Drawing upon the Noh narrative structure, Ishimure's work lay bare the precarious lives of marginalized humans, nonhumans, and other-than-humans, making precariousness visible.

As evident in the novel *Kugai jōdo,* Ishimure does not simply *document* the sufferings and struggles of those affected by Minamata disease but transforms their experiences into semi-fictional works. Ishimure does so in part to protect the sufferers' privacy (changing identifiable attributes), but also in order to make the sufferers' experiences and their world available to readers. Ishimure's semi-fictional, mythopoetic style conveys her subjects' experiences in a manner accessible to modern readers whose own experiences may not include concourse with the world of spirits.

Facilitating the sense of enmeshment of dual worlds in Ishimure's work, the identity of the narrator sometimes merges with that of the sufferers, as in *Kugai jōdo*. Here the perspective of the narrator is collapsed into that of the sufferer; the omniscient narrator descends to take on the point of view of the marginalized person "on the ground." This technique thereby invites the reader, whose perspective had been that of the god's eye view, into the sufferers' world. This collapse of the boundaries separating narrator from character and readers from sufferer indicates something of the ontology of a world otherwise, for it situates the reader-sufferer within an assemblage of humans and something other-than-human. In this way, Ishimure acts as a sort of medium: she oversees concourse between the modern world and the enspirited world of the marginalized. As Ishimure's works emphasize, despite differences in their constitutions, the two worlds are, after all, not mutually exclusive but overlapping, shared, interpenetrating.

I hasten to add one more point before examining Ishimure's work in depth. Ishimure's mythopoetic writing does not deny reality or function as a form of escapism. On the contrary, Ishimure portrays an enchanted world where humans, nonhumans, and other-than-humans build and maintain relationships. Her work functions not to divert from reality, but to invite readers into the reality of the world as a conglomerate of assemblages—a world enriched by recognition of our interconnection with those who are too often rendered invisible by the exclusionary forces of modernity.

NOH PLAYS, GENIUS LOCI, AND THE MERGING OF WORLDS

Like Noh plays, Ishimure's works make visible those who are usually invisible: the spirits and the marginalized. Noh took shape in the fourteenth century, deriving from Shinto rituals of song and dance dedicated to the deities.[9] In 2001, the United Nations Educational, Scientific, and Cultural Organization (UNESCO) designated Noh as an important form of cultural heritage leading to it being officially registered on the Representative List of the Intangible Cultural Heritage of Humanity in 2008.[10] The main character in Noh plays, especially in the Mugen Noh genre, is called a *shite* and is most often marginalized or other-than-human.[11] The supporting character, or *waki*, is a traveler, often a Buddhist monk. In Mugen Noh, these two characters encounter and converse—an intersection of this world and a world otherwise.

In the first act, the waki embarks on a journey and comes across a person on his route who shares knowledge of local history. After an intermission, the second act opens with the waki asleep. The shite appears in the waki's dream and narrates the shite's story in dance. After the story is recounted, the waki wakes and finds that the shite has disappeared.[12] The shite's story can only be told when the waki listens to the shite. In this regard, the waki serves as a mediating figure; the waki's willingness to listen to the story makes the shite and her story visible.

In order to represent the multidimensionality of the world otherwise that it portrays, the Noh stage features a bridge crossed by the shite, connecting the spirit world to the waki's locale. Bruce Allen explains the role of the bridge in Noh as follows: "The interaction of these elements [dance, music, narration, sounds, and motion] takes place in a mythopoetic space, or cosmology, that is created when one passes over a 'bridge' on a stage that links the worlds of reality and dreams, and the times of past, present, and future."[13] In an analogous manner, Ishimure's works conjure spaces where two worlds meet. In turn, her books themselves serve as bridges by which readers encounter a world otherwise.

Consider, for example, the famous Noh play *Izutsu*, written by a fourteenth/fifteenth-century Noh actor and playwright Zeami, also known as Kanze Motokiyo.[14] *Izutsu* begins on an autumn day, when a monk stops at Ariwara temple on his way to Hase temple in Yamato (present-day Nara) to pray for the dead spirits of a ninth-century aristocrat and poet, Ariwara Narihira, and his wife, to whom the temple was dedicated. A local woman comes by and begins to draw water from a well on the temple's grounds. She then turns to the monk and tells him how Narihira courted many women but, in the end, developed a true love for the woman with whom he grew up playing around the well, by which they stand. Narihira then devoted himself to this woman and took her as his wife. After the local woman finishes her story, she confides to the monk that she is that woman—Narihira's wife and daughter of Aritsune. The second act begins with the monk's decision to hold a memorial service for Narihira's wife. That night, the woman appears in his dream, dances in Narihira's robe, and seeks Narihira's reflection in the well. Eventually, the night ends, the woman disappears, and the monk wakes up from the dream.

It is significant that this story of the shite—Narihira's deceased wife—is told at the well, a place about which she and Narihira share fond memories. The well is the play's *topos*—a specific site where an event takes place, generating a story. According to theater critic Tsuchiya Keiichirō, narratives in Noh plays often follow a person's physical and emotional journey. During this journey, the waki approaches the mnemonically rich topos, a place that brings at the intersection of past and present, dream and reality, and this world and a world otherwise.[15] In Noh plays, the power of place is personified in the shite, the genius loci.

This power of place is also evident in Ishimure's work.[16] Not only in her Noh plays (she wrote two) but in novels like *Lake of Heaven* the genius loci is prominent. The novel tells the story of a young man, Masahiko, a composer who, finding himself unable to create music, experiences a loss of identity. He visits his grandfather Masahito's hometown, Amazoko (literally translated as "the bottom of Heaven"), for the first time, only to find that the village in which Masahito grew up has been submerged beneath the reservoir of a dam.[17] Like the Buddhist monk in a Noh play, Masahiko takes a journey from Tokyo—modern society—to a rural place redolent of an earlier era. Masahiko's encounter with the displaced villagers, including two women shamans, now living near the dam, bridges the modern world of Masahiko and the world of the former villagers, while also linking the present to the past. Listening to the villagers' stories about their coexistence with the spirit of various spots in the village, Masahiko regains his sense of identity, feeling anchored to those stories—not only as a composer but also as a grandson and member of the village. No longer experiencing himself as a discrete individual but as part of an assemblage. He returns to Tokyo, his ability to compose restored and his world enriched. *Lake of Heaven* is thus the story of the emergence of the two worlds in the character of Masahiko, the waki on his journey. Much as in a Noh play, the audience hears the story of a shite as received by the waki, in this novel, the reader learns the story of the spirits of Amazoko through the former villagers, as heard by Masahiko.

Amazoko village represents this world of the spirit—it no longer exists on the map, but it does live on in the villagers' stories. According to literary scholar

Matsuya Rie, what is valuable to the Amazoko villagers is not the "dignified Shinto shrine or the peaks of high mountains" that the tourists admire, but rather a nameless "weeping cherry tree" or an ordinary "moon shadow bridge" because these everyday places are so many facets of the villagers' relations to the village's topos. Such relations, sustained by stories, constitute the assemblages of which the villagers are a part.[18] Ishimure describes her vision of "the world" of assemblages—a world otherwise: "What I mean by 'the world' does not mean something translatable to cartography, but the world where all the beings, such as the grass on the beach, animals, and mountain deities, are fully alive. All of them interact with one another. When the mountain, water, river, and people's lives are healthy, they together produce a new story every day. Such a world is, in short, the world of the spirit."[19]

ENVIRONMENTAL REFUGEES AND THE DISCOURSE OF "HOME"

Now that we have established the importance of place, the land, topos, and the genius loci in Ishimure's work, I wish to discuss how this work may be read as a critique of the rhetoric of "home" as it is deployed in the discourse around Fukushima. The Japanese government has been campaigning for people to return to Fukushima by normalizing high radiation levels, hosting the Olympics,[20] and using propagandistic rhetoric such as "*fukkō*" (restoration), "*kizuna*" (bonding), and "*furusato*" (home/town). In this context, aspects of the importance of place that we have been examining are exploited to encourage the public to accept the government's policies. Reading Ishimure's works with this matter in mind will allow us to distinguish her understanding of furusato from the government's use of this term according to its agenda, with its accompanying exaltation of self-sacrifice. As we will see, Ishimure's furusato names a place free of self-sacrifice.

Rather than focusing on questions of what constitutes relatively "safe" levels of radiation—a matter beyond the scope of this project—I will critically examine policy rhetoric surrounding Fukushima, considering in particular how it is reminiscent of governmental rhetoric around Minamata. After the explosion and meltdown of the nuclear reactors at Fukushima on March 11, 2011, the Japanese government declared a state of emergency. It implemented a limited evacuation plan that left many people behind in Fukushima, living in an environment with a radiation level of 20 millisieverts (mSv) per year—twenty times higher than the national and international standards. Before the meltdown, the measurement of 20 mSv per year was only observed in adult male workers who dealt with nuclear materials, such as researchers in radiation laboratories and nuclear plant workers. Elevating the standard of allegedly safe radiation exposure encouraged citizens to stay in or to return to the affected area.

Following the earthquake and tsunami on March 11, evacuation orders had been issued for those living within a three-kilometer radius of the nuclear site; the next day, the radius was extended to ten kilometers. Then three reactors exploded, spewing radiation into the air. In April 2011, the Fukushima prefectural government divided the evacuated area into three zones which were given the following names, awkward in Japanese and even more so in English: the Difficult-to-Return Zone, the Restricted Residence Zone, and the Evacuation Order Cancellation Preparation Zone.[21] By 2017, most evacuation orders aside from Difficult-to-Return Zone were lifted; as of 2020, some parts of the Difficult-to-Return Zone are also accessible. However, the government has not yet rescinded the state of emergency. A policy that encourages people to stay in, or return to, an environment whose safety standard differs significantly from that of the rest of the country amounts to an act of violence, especially for a vulnerable population that includes pregnant women and children—yet this fact is rarely a point of discussion in public discourse around Fukushima.[22]

In treating the problems around these evacuation policies, I refer to people who would typically be called "evacuees" or "voluntary evacuees" (*jishu hinansha*) as "environmental refugees," so as to underscore the violence of the policies and the precarity produced by them. "Voluntary evacuees" is the name customarily attached to the people who, though living outside the designated evacuated zone, decided to leave. But this epithet suggests that the choice to evacuate is solely the responsibility of the individual, as indicated in the phrase *jiko sekinin*, or "one's own responsibility," which circulates widely as part of the government's rhetorical response to the crisis, even before this accident. I do not wish to criticize those who stayed behind in Fukushima: the decision to leave cannot be made solely by individual, despite the rhetoric of *jiko sekinin*, as we have already established the idea of independent and autonomous individuals as a modern myth. I additionally believe that those who stayed and those who left were purposefully divided against each other by the government, thereby impeding the ability to cooperate in seeking compensation, assignation of responsibility, and the like.

With these points in mind, I argue that the interaction with the genius loci advocated by Ishimure's invocation of furasato must not be misinterpreted and collapsed into the propagandistic discourse of "home." Indeed, Ishimure's furusato may be read as a critique of "homeland" as deployed by the state of Japan and its avid supporters in post-Fukushima discourse.

By leaving Fukushima behind, the environmental refugees inevitably felt uprooted; for some, Fukushima was their birthplace, and, for others, it was where they had established their families. With the rhetoric of furusato circulating in commercials, newspaper articles, and television shows, some refugees experience guilt for "abandoning" their hometown when they should have remained behind to work toward its restoration (fukko). By the same token, this rhetoric functioned to foster in those who stayed in Fukushima, a sense of pride for contributing to fukko and remaining in furusato—the homes and communities established on land inherited from their ancestors.

Thus, the word furusato not only evokes nostalgia but also contains moral valences; it conveys loyalty to one's hometown and filial piety in attending to the graves of, and land inherited from, one's ancestors; care for one's (extended) family. Holding on to such values, particularly during a time of crisis, may appear heroic to some. For example, the popular song *Furusato*, endorsed by the Ministry of Education for a century, is still widely sung in Japan, perhaps more so in the wake of March 11, 2011. Its nostalgic lyrics—the first verse of which conjures the mountains where one chased rabbits and the rivers where one caught small carp—closely link furusato with childhood memories and a strong sense of place. The second verse concerns the parents and friends whom one has not seen for a long time but who anchor one in the furusato. In the final verse, furusato is presented as a place in which one does not currently reside, but to which one will eventually return.

The song's popularity is attributed to the demographical shift, triggered by the regime change. The 1868 Meiji Restoration saw the beginning of political, educational, and economic centralization, with many youths drawn from their childhood furusato and into cities as college students, menial workers, or corporate employees. The mobility still continues to this day. A widespread sense of nostalgia among those who had left their rural homes found expression in the song *Furusato* when it was released in 1904. But this song does not reflect an innocent experience of a hometown idyll. Attention to the historical context from which the song emerged reveals that running after rabbits, far from the innocent pastime of frolicking children, was in fact encouraged as part of war efforts of the time. Scholar and philosopher Uchiyama Takashi observes that *Furusato* was released the year of the outbreak of the Russo-Japanese War. That war increased the demand for fur, which was needed to line soldiers' uniforms; many Japanese soldiers were not used to the subfreezing temperatures of Northeast China and Siberia, and the severe weather was debilitating. The Japanese Empire responded to the fur shortage by encouraging children to catch rabbits and donate the fur for the linings of uniforms.[23] Furusato—both the term and the song of that title—was closely linked to the nation's agenda—in this case, colonialism.

Let us now turn to Ishimure's usage of furusato.[24] Given the importance of genius loci in her works, Ishimure may appear to endorse the nostalgia of furusato—of staying in or returning to one's homeland. But a more nuanced reading reveals that her use of the word carries complex connotations not bound to the political agenda of promoting allegiance to, or forced residence within, an unsafe place. In her astute analysis of *Tenko*, Matsuya argues that Ishimure is opposed to exploitation of nostalgia toward (self-)sacrifice. Matsuya writes that "what Ishimure attempts to retrieve [from the submerged village] is the village's collective life, in which residents embraced mountain deities and sea deities, the collective history as well as each villager's personal history. This very place, holding all those memories within, is, in a word, *furusato* or homeland (hometown)."[25] Furusato contains memories, which also generate stories that foster collective ties. By Matsuya's reading of Ishimure, furusato, is not, or not only, a physical locale, but the memories and spirits of a place, which may be conveyed through stories. In this way, one need not reside in one's furusato in order to partake of its world otherwise. Furusato, in Ishimure's literature, is connected with, but not bound to, land; "home" may be experienced as a mythic space accessible through stories.

Matsuya argues that Ishimure's furusato does not necessarily point to the actual geographical location of one's birthplace or dwelling place but rather to this mythic space. Drawing upon the philosopher Yi-Fu Tuan's thoughts on the landscape, Matsuya elaborates on her point: Tuan writes, in a chapter entitled "Attachment to Homeland," that it is hardly imaginable for one to abandon one's homeland because one's "homeland" is the center of the world, or the universe, and therefore is the most meaningful place. What he refers to as "the center of the world; does not point to a certain place on the map but rather indicates a mythic concept."[26] Furusato may exist in memory and as a "mythic concept"; it is not something to be "restored," as fukko propaganda would have it, but imaginatively recreated in shared stories.

Furusato is the center of one's world precisely because it embraces and nurtures one. If furusato is the mythic center of the world, it cannot be physically restored. For those who, in accord with the propagandistic notion of homeland, remain or return to Fukushima, the false hopes of fukko are paid for with self-sacrifice in the form of radiation exposure—a risk higher than the rest of the country.

Ishimure believes not in the power of imposed self-sacrifice but in the power of story; indeed, she wields this power in her work. But she is also careful in her application of it. Literary scholar Toyosato Mayumi asserts that "Ishimure's narrative reveals how the discourse of home [*furusato*] affects a place and its social relationships and, moreover, its ambiguity: while it can be a frame for one's attachment to a familiar place and sense of locality to be expressed and heard, it may shackle one's subjectivity and its ethical autonomy."[27] The value of Ishimure's work lies in part in its ability to reveal the dangers and possibilities of furusato. In my reading of Ishimure, the mythic furusato she condones bears out the agency of assemblages rather than the agency of independent and autonomous entities.

Taken as a mythic realm rather than a literal homeland, Ishimure's furusato exerts no force that binds one or compels one to return to it; it makes no demand to remain in a place that might be harmful to one's health. Rather, Ishimure's mythopoetic writings foster the cultivation of a comparably mythopoetic sensibility in her readers—a sensibility by which one is free from geographical bounds and nostalgic bindings. Ishimure's personal experiences in Minamata fostered this mythic but antinostalgic sense of furusato. Eschewing romanticizing construals of "premodern" rural life, such as perpetuated by the nation's use of furusato, Ishimure recalls the social divisions that caused strife in her hometown as well as the marginalization of many of its residents—fishers, undertakers, and prostitutes. At the same time, Ishimure's use of furusato, which accommodates and disseminates the stories of those marginalized people, promotes an ethics of assemblage—a mythopoetic intercourse of, between, and among the precarious, whether humans, nonhumans, or other-than-humans.

Toyosato cites scholar of Japanese literature Karen Thornber in further explaining the complexity of Ishimure's notion of furusato. "Thornber regards some representations of the human/nonhuman symbiotic relationships and those of the sea as the local fishermen's 'home' or 'garden' in the novel as rather problematic in the sense that they mystify anthropocentric attitudes as well as the human impact on the environments." However, as Toyosato observes, "When seen from the viewpoint of literary convention, Ishimure's narrative, in contrast, works to defamiliarize the very discourse of home and leads us into a reconsideration of such a cultural framework."[28] As Toyosato insightfully argues, Ishimure's work undoes the anthropocentrism of the modern secular worldview, in which humans are set apart from, and often placed above, animals, even as it excludes other-than-humans. Her deployment of furusato neither mystifies anthropocentrism nor indulges in nostalgia. It thus makes itself "useless" to the propagandistic discourse of national "homeland" as well.

Indeed, Ishimure's furusato, far from reinforcing the nostalgic and nationalistic underpinnings of the national furusato discourse, enables one better to discern, and therefore reject, the demand for self-sacrifice under the guise of moral codes, and to cultivate a mythical notion of furusato to counter the physical and psychological constraints of the government's coercive rhetoric of "home." Indeed, Christine L. Marran, a scholar of Japanese literature and culture, compares the mythical sensibility of Ishimure's furusato to the process of decolonization; freeing oneself from the rhetorical power of this world resembles emancipation from the colonial appeals to homeland. Marran writes that "Ishimure's decolonial imagination rejects the claims of the self-indulgent national collectivity that silences critical voices within that presumed collectivity."[29] Ishimure's deep-seated concerns about the modern state's coercive, expansionist impulses give rise to a counternarrative of furusato that finds moral wisdom in the stories and perspectives of those whose lives are rendered precarious by colonial logics.

To be sure, Ishimure's resistance to the temptation to succumb to the power of the national agenda of "home"—with its gratifying nostalgia and romantic idealizations of place—was fostered by her interactions with those who were not welcomed in their geographical places of furusato. In response, Ishimure creates, or co-creates with those in states of precarity, a mythical realm, a safe space in which they may reside. Toyosato's analysis illuminates this point. Toyosato suggests that "the search for an alternative way of mapping Minamata is part of Ishimure's efforts to move beyond the discourse of home and to rewrite what comprises Minamata, and its relation to larger areas of Japan."[30] Toyosato further limns Ishimure's resistance:

> "Home" will forever remain a nostalgic *future*, pasted within and without with beautiful, if somewhat blurred and discolored photographs. If we could distance ourselves at equal distance from those who left home and those who, while still living in their native place, are compelled to leave it either in imagination or from time to time in reality, as the other members of the community in which they were born no longer allow them to call their home a real "home," we would perhaps be able to understand and appreciate a number of basic things: the real nature of the locality we call "home" or, in a broader context, of our native country; . . . Further, we would be able to perceive, or at least have a foretaste, [of] the hazy, abstract world of the future.[31]

Furusato enriches life not through restoration of a physical place to conform to an idealized past, but through stories that, fostering cultivation of a mythic sensibility, offer imaginations of a more equitable future in a world otherwise, however hazily conceived. Furusato, for Ishimure, is a world with no center, and thus no margins—a web of interconnections and intermingling forces.

Thus Ishimure does not criticize furusato as such, but rather, she challenges us to ponder whether the co-creation of furusato might contribute to an awareness of the precarity by which some lives may go unmourned.

Noh scholar Masuda Shōzō emphasizes that the presence of the waki enables the audience to visualize the interaction between two worlds: "In Mugen Noh, when the waki serves as a mediator by encountering a shite, an other-worldly being, the waki functions as *awai* (betweenness) and bridges the reality of this world and the imagination of the other world. The shite's strong emotions are only transformed from grudge to gratitude after having its voice heard by the waki."[32] Here, we see a similar structure in Ishimure's works. A character in her literature listens to the voice of other-than-humans as the waki in Noh play. Readers of her works as well as audience of Noh play experiences two worlds encounter and unfld in front of their eyes.

This is not to say that the experiences of Minamata sufferers or other tragic events must take the form of fiction or fantasy, but only to say that when the sufferers' raw emotions are generated from their experiences of rejection by, and alienation from, this world, understanding their plight requires a new frame through which to recognize their precarity. Tsuchiya's analysis of the Noh drama, too, resonates with Ishimure's work: "Humans become free from the narrative plot through the deconstruction and reconstruction of the story observed in a Noh play. Therefore, a Noh play is an art for liberation. Zeami and other Noh playwrights [in the medieval period] chose as protagonists the marginalized, women, and those who were discriminated against. By doing so, a Noh play tries to deconstruct [the norms and hierarchy of] a given society and its narrative."[33] Cultivating our mythic sensibilities and the ability to endure ambiguities in multiple worlds would free us from constraints, and thereby show more possibilities. This process is, at once, one of decolonizing oneself and of opening oneself to a world otherwise. In this sense, one could free oneself from the physical constraint of furusato, but open oneself to a mythic realm of furusato that nurtures one.

Bruce Allen rightly calls Ishimure a "modern mythmaker." I believe that we require new myths and new ways of mythmaking. According to Allen, Ishimure "insist[s] that it is both possible and essential to create new myths through modern forms of storytelling."[34] Such myths would offer models for alternative ways of being in this world, and being at home in the world. New myths such as envisioned by Ishimure will help us to realize a furusato—or many "homes"—in which lives are valued rather than exploited, and in which moral imperatives do not demand self-sacrifice from among a precarious population. As English writer John Berger writes, "Never again will a single story be taken as though it is the only one,"[35] new imaginings of furusato will generate and accommodate pluralities of stories rather than enabling the domination and dominion of a single story.

What we need now is not simply to replace one myth with another but rather to learn how to navigate ourselves among multiple myths and worlds. Such plurality of perspectives—with multiple agencies, empathies, and emotional investments—might help redress conditions of exploitation in which self-sacrifice is glorified. Thus attuning ourselves to multiplicities that embrace, rather than exploit, the marginal and care for, rather than coerce, the precarious humans, animals, and others who are assembled therein will enable "a notion of publics as human-nonhuman collectives that are provoked into existence by a shared experience of harm."[36] Much like the Noh plays that inform her literature, Ishimure seeks to bring about a world otherwise, a world that is not a single or singular world.

NOTES

1. The Burj Khalifa, a residential and commercial building in Dubai in the United Arab Emirates, exceeds the height of the Sky Tree by over 200 meters.

2. Masuo, Shin'ichirō, and Joseph P. Elacqua, "Chinese Religion and the Formation of Onmyōdō," *Japanese Journal of Religious Studies* 40, no. 1 (2013): 29. This article by Masuo and Elacqua suggests that the jichinsai, translated by them as *land-quelling ritual*, was performed by Onmyōji in the late eighth century. On occasions when Buddhist organizations erect new buildings, however, a Buddhist priest conducts a similar ritual to pacify the earth spirit according to their tradition.

3. Kobayashi, Toshiyuki, "Nihonjin no shūkyōteki ishiki ya kōdō wa dou kawattaka—ISSP Kokusai hikaku chōsa 'Shūkyō' Nihon no kekka kara" (How have Japanese religious thoughts and behaviors changed—ISSP [International Social Survey Programme] international comparative studies on 'Religion' a case of Japan), *Hōsō kenkyū to chōsa* 69, no. 4 (2019): 53.

4. When Tsu city in Mie prefecture commissioned a jichinsai from Shinto priests with a 4,000-yen honorarium in 1965, a city official Sekiguchi Seiichi who was asked to attend the ceremony, together with over hundred guests. Sekiguchi found that it was a violation of separation of the state and religion, as is stated in the Japanese Constitution, article 20 (3): "The State and its organs will not engage in any religious education or any other religious activity." Sekiguchi filed a charge against the mayor of Tsu city, who was tried at the local court and, in a higher court and, finally, in the supreme courts. Ultimately, on July 13, 1977, the supreme court concluded that "the ceremony did not promote Shinto or raise Shinto consciousness among the average person," and, thus, "the government did not engage in a religious activity in violation of the constitution." Brent T. White, "Reexamining Separation: The Construction of Separation of Religion and State in Post-War Japan" *Pacific Basin Law Journal,* 22, no. 1 (2004): 40–42.

5. Bruce Allen, "Introduction" to Karen Thornber, "Ishimure Michiko and Global Ecocriticism," *The Asia-Pacific Journal* 14, no. 13 (6) (2016). 1.

6. Bruce Allen's introduction to Michiko Ishimure and Bruce Allen, "Secret Song," *World Literature Today* 82, no. 4 (2008): 31.

7. Yoko Kurahashi, "Creating a Tapestry of Voice and Silence in Michiko Ishimure's 'Kugai jōdo' (Paradise in the Sea of Sorrow)," *Journal of Narrative Theory* 33, no. 3 (2003): 326.

8. Bruce Allen, Introduction to *Lake of Heaven*, by Michiko Ishimure, trans. Bruce Allen (Lanham, MD: Rowman & Littlefield, 2008), xi.

9. Min Tian, "Chinese Nuo and Japanese Noh: Nuo's Role in the Origination and Formation of Noh," *Comparative Drama* 37 no. 3/4 (2003–2004): 343–360. In this chapter, I describe a Noh play as a Japanese traditional play, but Min Tian has studied Noh's origin and traces it to the Chinese exorcism rite, Nuo.

10. Sugisawa, Haruko, "Noh no monogurui ni tsuite no kenkyū" (A study of "Monogurui Noh"), *Yūgō bunka kenkyū* 7 (2006): 66.

11. Shite is conventionally categorized into the following five types: a deity, a dead male person, a dead female person, a mentally disturbed person, or an *oni* (ogre).

12. Masuda, Shōzō, *Zeami no sekai* (The world of Zeami) (Tokyo: Shūeisha, 2007), 46.

13. Bruce Allen, "The Noh Imagination in Shiranui and the Work of Ishimure Michiko," in *Ishimure Michiko's Writing in Ecocritical Perspective: Between Sea and Sky*, ed. Bruce Allen and Yuki Masami (Lanham, MD: Rowman & Littlefield, 2008), 175.

14. He was born into a family of Noh players headed by Kan'ami and learned to dance at an early age. The most powerful man of the time, Ashikaga Yoshimitsu, the third shogun of Ashikaga shogunate, discovered his talent. Thanks to Ashikaga's patronage, the Noh play became a popular art form catering to commoners as well as a sophisticated art form for aristocrats and the warrior class.

15. Tsuchiya, Keiichirō, *Noh: Dorama ga tachiarawareru toki* (Noh: When a drama emerges) (Tokyo: Kadokawa, 2014), 14.

16. Ishimure also wrote two Noh plays of her own. One is *Shiranui* (2002), which was first played in July 2002 at Hōshō Nohgakudō and Kokuritsu Nohgakudō, followed by Kumamot prefectural hall in August 2003, and at Eco Park in Minamata in August 2004, and again in Tokyo in October. Watanabe, *Mouhitotsu no konoyo*, 118–119. Also see Karen Thornber, "Ishimure Michiko and Global Ecocriticism" *The Asia-Pacific Journal,* 14, no. 13 (6) (2016): 1–23. Another is *Okinomiya* (2018), set in Amakusa, triggered by 2001's triple disaster in Northern Japan. Shimura Fukumi and Ishimure Michiko, *Yuigon: taidan to oufukushokan* (The will: The dialogue and letters) (Tokyo: Chikuma shobō, 2014).

17. As we have seen in Ishimure's involvement in the trial where the members played with words ("shimin" with the character of death, or "Chisso" with the character of shame), the protagonist's name carries significance. Masa in Masahiko and Masahito indicates truth, righteousness, authenticity, while hiko means a (common) man and hito means a human.

18. Matsuya, Rie, "Kūkan no keiken to shite no fuukei: Yi-Fu Tuan kara Ishimure Michiko e" (Landscape as an Experience of Space: From Yi-Fu Tuan to Michiko Ishimure), *Kokusai Bunkagaku Kenkyū* 38 (2012): 14–15.

19. Ishimure, *Soseishita tamashii o nosete*, 162.

20. Softball and baseball games were planned to be held in Fukushima. In addition, as a preparation for the Olympics, the torch relay was to start in Fukushima. See Norma Field, "Introduction" of "This Will Still Be True Tomorrow: 'Fukushima Ain't Got the Time for Olympic Games': Two Texts on Nuclear Disaster and Pandemic," *The Asia-Pacific Journal,* 18, no. 13 (2) (2020): 1–10. Also, see Mathieu Gaulène, "Does the Advertising Giant Dentsu Pull the Strings of the Japanese Media?" trans. Sachie Mizohata, *The Asia-Pacific Journal,* 14, no. 11 (5) (2016). https://apjjf.org/2016/11/Gaulene.html. The Tokyo Olympics, originally scheduled to be held in 2020, was a part of the Fukushima restoration, as a few games of baseball and softball would have taken place. Antoni Slodkowski, Nathan Layne, Mari Saito, Ami Miyazaki, "$8.2 million by Tokyo Olympics bid lobbied figure at center of French corruption probe" *Reuters,* March 30, 2020. https://www.reuters.com/article/us-olympics-2020-lobbying-exclusive/exclusive-japan-businessman-paid-8-2-million-by-tokyo-olympics-bid-lobbied-figure-at-center-of-french-corruption-probe-idUSKBN21I0CX.

21. Fukushima Prefectural webpage: https://www.pref.fukushima.lg.jp/site/portal-english/en03-08.html.

22. Those who recognize violent acts are not resigned to them, however. One of the admirable attempts is *Kodomo datsu hibaku saiban,* or the Trial to Protect Children from Irradiation.

23. Such an association of furusato and nationalism is hardly new and is not specific to Japan, either. Historian George L. Mosse unpacks the close connection between war and the rhetoric of homeland by investigating the representations of nature—mountains and rivers—that elevated the protection of the mother/fatherland as a moral value among people in Germany during World War I and instigated the fervor for the war. George L. Mosse, *Fallen Soldiers: Reshaping the Memory of the World Wars* (New York: Oxford University Press, 1991).

24. Ogata, Masato, "Minamatbyō kara Fukushima genpatsujiko o kanngaeru: Gendai bunmei no futsugou na shinjitsu" (Think about the Fukushima nuclear accident from the viewpoint of Minamata disease: The inconvenient truth of modern civilization), *Tamashii utsure,* 48 (2012): 20. Ogata Masato, one of the founders of Hongan no kai and the main character examined in chapter 7, has an idea similar to Ishimure's on the notion of furusato, but Ogata uses the term *shōgoku,* literally meaning a country of birth, rather than furusato. However, as will be discussed, like Ishimure's furusato, Ogata's *shōgoku* designates a metaphysical and mythical place, not a geographical location.

25. Matsuya, "Kūkan no keiken to shite no fuukei," 12.

26. Matsuya, "Kūkan no keiken to shite no fuukei," 12.

27. Toyosato, Mayumi, "Mapping Nonmodernity: Home and the World in Ishimure Michiko's *Kugai jōdo,*" in *Ishimure Michiko's Writing in Ecocritical Perspective: Between Sea and Sky*, eds. by Bruce Allen and Yuki, Masami (Lanham, MD: Lexington Books, 2016), 63.

28. Toyosato, "Mapping Nonmodernity," 59.

29. Christine L. Marran, *Ecology without Culture: Aesthetics for a Toxic World* (Minneapolis, MN: University of Minnesota Press, 2017), 52.

30. Toyosato, "Mapping Nonmodernity," 67.

31. Toyosato, "Mapping Nonmodernity," 70. *Kugai jōōdo,* 376. Change made and shown in italics by Toyosato.

32. Masuda, *Zeami no sekai,* 26.

33. Tsuchiya, *Noh*, 8–9. In a broder conversation, Murakami Haruki discusses the relationship between tamashii and narratives: "Narratives, in short, reside deep in one's tamashii. They should be present there. It is because the narrative exists in the deepest bottom of one's tamashii, they are able to relate to one another." Murakami Haruki, *Shokugyō to shite no shōsetsuka* (*Novelist as a Vocation*) (Tokyo: Shinchōsha, 2015), 337. Translation mine.

34. Bruce Allen, "Facing the True Costs of Living," in *Coming into Contact: Explorations in Ecocritical Theory and Practice*, eds. Annie Merrill Ingram et al. (Athens, GA: University of Georgia Press, 2007), 161. Thomas A. Tweed's following sentences will also be helpful to consider the contribution of religious studies to this new environmental ethics of mythmaking: "I decided, however, that two other

orienting metaphors are most useful for analyzing what religion is and what it does: spatial metaphor (dwelling and crossing) signal that religion is about finding a lace and moving across space, and aquatic metaphors (confluences and flows) signal that religions are not reified substances but complex processes." Thomas A. Tweed, *Crossing and Dwelling: A Theory of Religion* (Cambridge, MA: Harvard University Press, 2006), 59.

35. John Berger, *G* (New York: Vintage Books, 1972), 133.

36. Bennett, *Vibrant Matter,* xix.

Chapter 7

Hongan no Kai and Spiritual Praxis as an Environmental Ethics

In August 1996, two committees of Minamata sufferers and supporters—one based in Minamata and one in Tokyo—were collaborating in preparation for an exhibition at a special hall in front of JR Shingawa station in Tokyo, scheduled for September 28 through October 13. The exhibition comprised 300 photos and 60 items showing the magnitude of methylmercury poisoning in Minamata. For the Minamata committee, the exhibition was an occasion not just for disseminating information about the disease; it was also a space for conveying the experiences of the sufferers and for mourning those who had died from the poisoning by inviting their tamashii into the exhibition space.

Ogata Masato, who sat on the Minamata committee, therefore decided to sail from the reclaimed land of Minamata to Tokyo in his wooden sailboat, commonly referred to as an *utasebune*. If the photos at the exhibition aimed to inform visitors of the plight that originated from the methylmercury in Chisso's wastewater, Ogata believed it was his duty to bring the *tamashii*—specifically, the spirits of the departed, humans and nonhumans alike—with him to the exhibition. Nothing was more appropriate for this journey, thought Ogata, than departing from Minamata's *suigin bakushinchi,* or ground zero.

In light of the danger of the trip, Ogata's plan did not meet with unanimous support. Undertaking the 1,400-kilometer (870-mile) voyage from Minamata to Tokyo in a small wooden boat would be perilous. Later recalling his journey, Ogata acknowledged the risks: the four masts were disproportionately tall for the boat's size, which made the boat susceptible to winds that could topple it; the engine was old, and it could have broken down at any moment; and the boat's hull was fragile, its wood disintegrating. Indeed, water seeped into the boat a few times while Ogata was sailing.[1]

Persuaded by Ogata's firm determination, his friends and supporters finally embraced the plan. Ishimure Michiko was among them, naming Ogata's boat *Nichigetsumaru* (The Sun and the Moon).[2] With wishes for Ogata's safe travel, Ishimure and her fellow Hongan no kai members hosted a *shukkongi* ceremony (a ritual for invoking tamashii) to see Ogata and the *Nichigetsumaru* off from Minamata's reclaimed land on the night of August 13. Alongside the Hongan no kai members, eighty other attendees from Tokyo, Fukuoka, Kumamoto, and Minamata gathered for the ceremony.[3]

Meanwhile, members of the exhibition committees in Tokyo and Minamata were engaged in heated debate. The Tokyo committee had solicited ideas from those in Minamata for holding an inaugural event the night before the exhibition's opening. Responding to the Tokyo committee's call, Ishimure proposed that the Tokyo group hold its own shukkongi. Ishimure and Minamata sufferers would travel to Tokyo to attend the ceremony, donning white robes to set fire to the debris of the *Nichigetsumaru*'s disassembled parts—a gesture to welcome the tamashii off the boat. According to Ishimure, this ritual would bring together the spirits of the dead—not just people, but all beings—cats, fish, seaweed, and any others—that had suffered methylmercury poisoning from Chisso's wastewater. But upon hearing Ishimure's proposal, many of the Tokyo committee members found the idea of the ceremony repugnant; it appeared too "religious" to them. Despite Ishimure's thorough explanation of the ritual's significance and the Minamata committee's intentions, the Tokyo committee declined to attend the shukkongi, and even considered withdrawing from the exhibition altogether.

Sociologist Kurihara Akira, one of the Tokyo committee's chief members, recalled with regret the Tokyo committee's response. When the committee objected to the shukkongi's religious nature, Kurihara argued that the ritual was not religious in a general sense since it was not affiliated with any organized religious institution. Thus, he claimed, participating in the shukkongi would not promote any particular religious belief. But more importantly, continued Kurihara in defense of the ritual, the shukkongi was a manifestation of the Minamata sufferers' worldview, displaying their fellowship with other beings—humans, nonhumans, and other-than-humans.

As Kurihara asserted, the shukkongi was also a way for the sufferers to question the values of a world that had delegitimized human solidarity with nonhumans and other-than-humans—an attitude that the Tokyo committee had now inadvertently displayed. Thus, in turning down the shukkongi proposal, the Tokyo committee members also rejected the Minamata committee members' worldview. Ultimately, the debate resulted in the Tokyo committee deciding not to support the ritual, but allowing individual members to assist in the shukkongi.

Kurihara found this whole incident surrounding the shukkongi proposal highly unsettling; after all, the Tokyo committee had solicited ideas for the exhibition's opening event, yet it had resisted the shukkongi plan. The Tokyo committee's concerns emerged against the background of an event that occurred only a year before the planned exhibition. A religious group—often referred to in the popular press as a "cult"—called Aum Shinrikyō had released sarin gas in crowded cars on three Tokyo subway lines, resulting in the deaths of fourteen people and injuries to more than six thousand. This incident promoted increasing aversion to religion among the people of Japan, who had already grown wary of religion following the World War II. During the war, Shinto, long associated with worship of the emperor, had been widely espoused as part of a virulent nationalism. This nationalistic fervor motivated reckless military operations and coerced suicide attacks from kamikaze pilots and torpedo crews, even as thousands of Japanese people in battle and at home died premature deaths by starvation. The Japanese Empire's invasions and colonial-expansionist endeavors were justified under the banner of *seisen*— "holy war."

Even in light of this fraught history of religion and violence in Japan, Kurihara still wondered why the Tokyo committee felt that including a religious ceremony as part of the exhibition was so problematic—especially when the ceremony had no affiliation with any specific religious organization. Moreover, the Minamata committee had repeatedly affirmed that it had no intention to advocate for the particular beliefs of any religious institution. Recognizing that the shukkongi would thus adhere to no religious doctrine, Kurihara was prompted to ask himself where this adamant refusal of the ritual came from.[4]

The Tokyo committee's response calls to mind the Danish cartoon controversy that we briefly touche in chapter 5.[5] We noted there that Saba Mahmood laments the press' framing of the incident, according to a reductive dichotomy between "secular" liberals, who value freedom of expression, and some religious communities, which do not share, or even reject, this value. Too often, Mahmood observes, the attitudes of religious communities are interpreted as backward and intolerant in this dichotomized framework. Mahmood's argument in her essay may make one realize the mechanism of precarity, for the harm done to religious communities—in this case, Muslim communities in Europe and beyond—is not treated in a manner commensurate with harm done on the basis of sex, gender, or race. Rather, Muslims and others who voiced "moral injury" were further ridiculed as uncivilized and irrational by those representing modern "secular" values.

According to this "secular" worldview, religion is perceived as a choice—to believe or not to believe, to belong or not to belong. Thanks to this framing of religion as a choice, Mahmood asserts, the ECHR did not take up the case of moral injury to Muslims. Yet, the ECHR had tried other cases involving perceived offenses to "Christian sensibilities," protecting "against seriously offensive attacks on matters regarded as sacred by Christians."[6] In her analysis of the Danish cartoon controversy, Mahmood reveals that the European legal system—supposedly representing secular ideals—is neither neutral nor impartial but, rather, heavily oriented toward protecting the Christian sensibility.[7] Moreover, secular individuals and institutions fail to realize, or do not admit to realizing, their own religious biases when labeling others as religious and, therefore, as irrational.[8]

Concurring with Mahmood, William Rasch criticizes German writer, artist, and public intellectual Günter Grass, who viewed the Danish cartoon controversy in terms of secular liberals versus religious fundamentalists. Although Grass assumes that fundamentalists are found not just among Muslims but also Christians and other religious traditions, Rasch interprets that Grass asserts that nonfundamentalists are the ones who shared the value stemming from "the Renaissance and the Enlightenment" and who thus enjoy "presumably higher or more advanced level of development." What nonfundamentalists should do, according to Grass, is to respect and tolerate the nonfundamentalist other.[9]

Arguing against Grass's view, Rasch observes that the Enlightenment tradition in Europe (and North America) determines what counts as secular, which is equated with "universal" and "neutral" rationalism and free of the "irrational" ideologies of religion. But as Rasch observers, the secular realm is not "neutral"—as the ECHR decisions mentioned above demonstrate.[10] "Secularism itself," Rasch argues, "with all its explicit assumptions about the political autonomy of citizens, the rational nature of the human being, and the disenchantment of politics to which autonomy is necessarily linked, remains the other of all [religious] worldviews."[11] Rasch further argues that secularism is a particular, rather than a universal, ideology, a belief system that liberals rely on to justify the espousal of liberalism's superiority over other worldviews.

In the case of the shukkongi debate ahead of the Minamata exhibition in Tokyo, Tokyo committee members who saw themselves as politically progressive to the extent of supporting the exhibition appear to have viewed religion as "backward" or associated it with a dangerous nationalism. The aforementioned historical exploitations of religion as part of a militaristic national agenda, as well as the recent Aum Shinrikyō terrorist attacks, surely colored Tokyo committee members' perception of religion, now linked with violence. On the one hand, I appreciate their caution toward religion, their attempt to avoid condoning beliefs that might be used to justify violence (such as found in the current revival of Shinto nationalism).[12] On the other hand, I also question secularism's supposed superiority and self-proclaimed rationality. Not defending religiously-motivated violence, I claim that secular nations and corporations have committed violence against humans and the environment at an unprecedented scale, with Minamata disease as well as the nuclear meltdown in Fukushima, epitomizing the harm caused by supposedly rational agents.

As we have seen, Ogata, Ishimure, and the Minamata committee members' belief in tamashii reflected their worldview. They believed the exhibition should invoke the presence of the victims' tamashii. Without the presence of the tamashii, the exhibition would be incomplete. Ogata, Ishimure, and the Minamata committee members were trying to not only exhibit the sheer horror of methylmercury poisoning but also to create an occasion for mourning the deceased and cultivating sympathy for sufferers. To that end, welcoming tamashii from afar and holding a ritual to express gratitude for their visit were indispensable. The disagreement between the two committees reveals their conflicting worldviews and identities: the Tokyo committee members regarded the shukkongi proposal as a threat to their secular identity as "progressive" citizens concerned with other people and the environment while being free of religion's "backward" and potentially dangerous beliefs.

In discussing some problems and contradictions in secularism, I am not calling for a return to religion. I am skeptical about religious beliefs that demand uncritical obedience and justify violence, just as I am skeptical of other belief systems that demand unquestioning obedience and justify violence, whether they come in the forms of nationalism and capitalism or under the guise of upholding the social norms of the majority, even at the expense of the continuing marginalization of those who do not fit within those norms. Yet, supposedly rational and ostensibly secular institutions, as the ECHR example makes clear, may fail to recognize and critique the less-than-rational aspects of its own belief systems. If the consequence of such supposed rationality is a system that produces precariousness, the "irrationality" of a world otherwise is surely preferable.

In considering the role that "irrational" practices might play in producing a world otherwise, this chapter addresses Hongan no kai's religious sensibility, as manifested in their ritual of carving stone bodhisattva statues—their way of engaging tamashii in attempting to realize a more just society. Hongan no kai's praxis, I wish to show, challenges secular rationalism in demonstrating an alternative way of building relationships with other beings and with one's natural surroundings. As we will see, the ritual act of carving statues and placing them on the reclaimed land of Minamata emerges alongside other sustainable practices among Minamata residents seeking alternative modes of living.

THE EMERGENCE OF HONGAN NO KAI

Hongan no Kai was founded in March 1994 with seventeen members, including Hamamoto Tsuginori, Taue Yoshiharu, Sugimoto Eiko and Takeshi,

Ogata Masato, Ishimure Michiko, and Kanazashi Junpei.[13] Kanazashi, originally from Shizuoka Prefecture, was not a Minamata native. However, upon graduating from college in Tokyo, he relocated to Minamata to join Minamata Seikatsu Gakkō, the Minamata School of the Art of Living (hereafter, Seikatsu Gakkō), established by Yanagida Kōichi. Although Yanagida was not a member of Hongan no kai, I will briefly discuss his activities, as Seikatsu Gakkō influenced Hongan no kai with its emphasis on collective, sustainable living.

Yanagida was born in Takuma, a village in Houtaku County (now part of Kumamoto City), Kumamoto Prefecture, in 1950. After graduating from Kumamoto Agricultural High School, he debated whether he should take over his family's business of rice and dairy farming or continue his education. His aspiration to attend university in a big city won out, and Yanagida became a student at Tokyo University of Agriculture in 1970. During this time, encouraged by his college friends, Yanagida joined his first sit-in in front of Chisso headquarters. After this experience, he participated in many more political demonstrations, mainly organized by Minamatabyō o kokuhatsu suru kai (the Association to indict [those responsible for] Minamata disease; see chapter 5).[14]

Yanagida devoted himself to Kokuhatsu suru kai's activities, to the extent that he eventually withdrew from his university studies. Moving back to Kumamoto, he undertook the role of organizer for Sōshisha, which was established in 1974, responding to the Minamata appeal that advocated for the establishment of the Minamatabyō sentā (Center for Minamata Disease) at the first United Nations Conference on the Human Environment in Stockholm.[15] Through Sōshisha's works, Yanagida set two missions: first, to experiment with an alternative, sustainable lifestyle; and, second, to disseminate the historical information concerning Minamata disease.

The first mission emerged from Yanagida's conviction that the modern lifestyle harms both humans and the environment. He defined this lifestyle in terms of *Chisso gata shakai,* or a "Chisso-type society" in which the system of mass production structures people's lives and shapes individuals' thoughts. As an antithesis to this Chisso-type society, Yanagida pursued a lifestyle that could enrich individual experiences through collective living, which he called a "Minamata-type society." Citizens in a Minamata-type society would seek a lifestyle less harmful to humans and the environment. Such a quest would need to be built upon knowledge about Minamata disease and its consequences.

In 1977, to fulfill his mission, Yanagida opened Minamata Jissen Gakkō (Minamata school of practice), where participants were trained to lead self-sustaining lives, learned farming and fishing from local Minamata residents, and educated themselves about Minamata disease while living collectively.

After five years, in 1982, the school changed its name to Minamata Seikatsu Gakkō, running for another decade before closing in 1992.

Kanazashi attended this school after having turned down several employment opportunities at corporations promising sufficient salaries for a comfortable life. Kanazashi recalls an episode toward the end of his student life at Jōchi University, where he majored in mechanical engineering. With his graduation approaching, Kanazashi visited his adviser to discuss his decision to move to Minamata after graduation. While this professor shared Kanazashi's long-standing concerns about environmental toxins and pollution-causing lifestyles, he said, "I have engaged in my research with a conviction that my study would contribute to the happiness of humankind. Now, we are facing dire situations of pollution and environmental destruction, but this is just a transitory phase, I believe. We will regain a more stable and safer environment [thanks to scientific research]." Facing his adviser, whose expertise lay in metallic materials for nuclear power reactors, Kanazashi merely uttered, "I cannot think in the same way you do."[16] Kanazashi could not share his adviser's optimistic belief in science and technology alone, creating a better environment for humans. Since migrating to Minamata, Kanazashi has produced washi, a traditional Japanese paper, which he learned to make at Seikatsu Gakkō. He opened his house for youths from Japan and beyond to attend workshops that he organizes. In these workshops, in addition to making washi, Kanazashi shares his knowledge and experiences in maintaining a sustainable lifestyle.

The idea of forming a group was already incubating in the minds of Kanazashi and Minamata sufferers before Hongan no kai's formation in 1994. In 1990, Kumamoto Prefecture finished burying the methylmercury residue that had accumulated in Minamata Bay after thirteen years of construction. The project revealed that more than half of the estimated 380 to 455 tons of methylmercury had either flowed into Minamata Bay or escaped into the air.[17] The completion of the land reclamation that had begun in 1977 made this pollution invisible, generating a sense among residents that the end of the Minamata incident was at hand. Following the land reclamation, beautification began. The land was covered with flowers, plants, and trails, and named Eco Park Minamata. Shared concerns that these aesthetic enhancements, administered by the municipal office, were intent on suppressing negative associations with the disease and thus diminishing the memory of the suffering it wrought, would bring together the seventeen people who then found Hongan no kai.

Minamata City, meanwhile, also sought to administer memory of the disease in its own way. The reclaimed and beautified land became the site of the Minamata Disease Museum, administered by the city. Although the museum narrates the history of the disease, it does not fulfill what Hongan no kai considers a vital aspect of commemorating the disease: maintaining intimacy with tamashii. The city also appropriated the phrase *moyai naoshi*—a phrase indicating a binding-together—in its appeal to residents. The phrase incorporates the fishing term *moyai,* which originally indicated the rope that ties a boat to shore, and the action of tying and mending or repairing broken bonds. The city launched the *Moyai Naoshi* campaign to restore trust in the government as well as relations among citizens who were sharply divided between fishers and Chisso workers, Minamata sufferers and non-sufferers. Despite these efforts to solidify the city's fragmented population, Hongan no kai members remained skeptical of the city's efforts; for them, relations with tamashii must be cared for in order to restore broken social and political relations. As a "secular" institution, the city made no provisions for tamashii.

Those who later became members were also concerned about these municipally initiated activities, feeling they might falsely convey that the crisis was over while none of the fundamental issues facing Minamata had been resolved. They also worried that all the feel-good additions to the city's history would conceal the plight of Minamata sufferers, allowing it to fade from people's minds. Sugimoto Takeshi thought it apparent that the concerned parties aside from the sufferers—Chisso, Minamata City, Kumamoto Prefecture, and the central government—wanted to put the outbreak in the past in order to present Minamata as a newly reborn, sanitized, toxin free, and environmentally conscious city. Following the completion of the land reclamation, a 1994 court decision ordering compensation for Minamata disease sufferers may have further given the public the false impression that Minamata disease was finally resolved. These concerns prompted some residents to voice their fears that the sufferings of Minamata residents would be forgotten.[18]

Thus a host of concerns around the memory of Minamata disease led to the formation of Hongan no kai. From its inception, this group sought ways to commemorate the disease and to develop alternative lifestyles oriented around avoiding another environmental catastrophe. In an interview with Ogata Masato, economist and ecologist Hara Takeshi asked Ogata why he had proposed the name *hongan*, when the word is associated with the Buddhist belief in Amida Buddha (Amitābha) of the Jōdo (Pure Land) and Jōdo-shin (True Pure Land) schools, prevalent in the Minamata region. In the context of the teachings of these schools, *hongan* refers to the vow for universal salvation made by Hōzō—the bodhisattva who would become the enlightened Amida Buddha. In reply, Ogata disclosed that despite its name, the group was not affiliated with, or aspiring to be, a religious entity. "The word *hongan* holds a religious connotation," but "we are not a religious organization."

The group's name is thus a critical appropriation of a Buddhist term for "vow," and therefore a way of invoking a sacred vow and carrying out its commitments—something that Ogata felt that both secular and religious institutions, including Buddhism, had failed to do. For its members, Hongan no kai's name also serves to remind people about the unsatisfactory outcome of the Chisso trial. "I have witnessed," continues Ogata, "many cases in which people's sufferings from Minamata disease are reduced only to political issues while its religious dimensions are left out. I was frustrated that the politics around Minamata disease alone was taken up and discussed in public, which prompted me to take a religious name for the group."[19] In the minds of Ogata and his fellow Hongan no kai members, if we are sincere about preventing a recurrence of Minamata, the discourse surrounding tamashii, genius loci, *funadama*, and *uo-don*—nonhuman and other-than-human beings, that is, who have not been regarded as having political agency—must be addressed alongside political and legal discussions.

Ogata further elaborates upon the religious innuendoes embedded in the group's name. For example, Ogata's household belonged to Nishi-Honganji, a denomination of the True Pure Land school, but none of his family members had been religious enough to declare faith in Amida Buddha in their everyday lives. Rather, they put their faith in funadama, the spirit of the boat, or in the fish and the sea. Later in his life, Ogata had an opportunity to learn about the teachings of Shinran—the founder of the True Pure Land school who was excommunicated from the mainstream Tendai school that devoted to the salvation of the aristocratic class. Shinran disobeyed the Tendai authority, disseminating Amida's teachings to commoners. Shinran's courage to stand against authority, and his firm determination to go his own way, appealed to Ogata. But Ogata, though inspired by Shinran's example, had less interest in scholastic debates around his teachings; he was interested in how Shinran's teachings might be enacted in everyday life. Ogata comments that instead of listening to a priest's lecture on Shinran's teachings, "I would rather ask a priest what he thinks of Minamata disease and the modern system [that caused it]."[20]

Ogata offered another elaboration when a True Pure Land priest whom he had known asked Ogata why he had named the group Hongan no kai. "By all rights," Ogata answered rather provocatively, "you should be upset with me for the fact that I used the name Hongan without consulting you. . . . It is a shame and you should not be pleased or be smiling to learn the name of our group. Why did I name the group Hongan no kai? Because you, priests, are not reliable."[21] The Buddhist temples in Minamata were silent not only about the suffering caused by the disease but also about Chisso's negligence. In its very name Hongan no kai was declaring its vow to respond to the problems and sufferings arising from Minamata disease, which Buddhism had ignored.[22]

However, choosing hongan as part of the group's name was not merely a reaction to institutional Buddhism. Ogata continued to unpack the meaning of the vow, as conceived apart from Amida's vow of universal salvation, with its rebirth in the "pure land." "Our objective," Ogata explains in a Hongan no kai newsletter, "is to deepen the notion of *inochi no negai,* or a 'vow for life.'"[23] Appreciating the lives of humans as well as nonhumans like fish and other sea creatures is not merely a theoretical moral doctrine; Ogata points to a reality in which one's life depends on many other lives within one's surroundings. Ogata, as a fisher, constantly reminds himself that such "appreciation" also

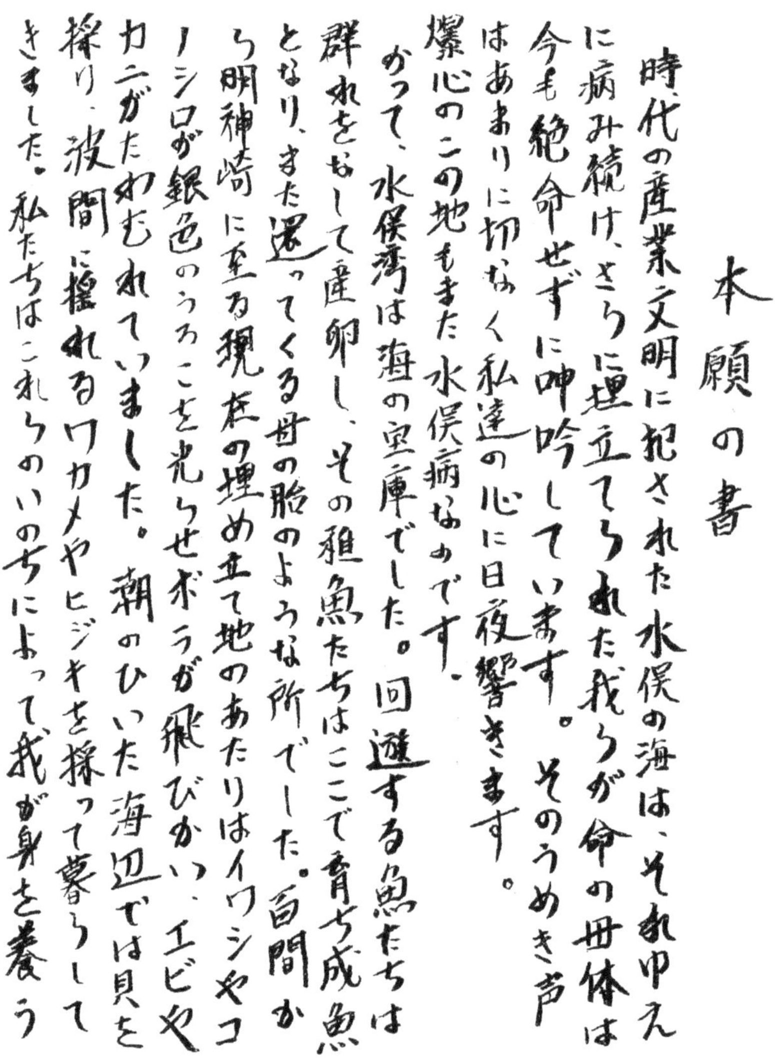
本願の書

時代の産業文明に犯された水俣の海は、それゆえに病み続け、さらに埋立てられた我らが命の母体は今も絶命せずに呻吟しています。そのうめき声はあまりに切なく私達の心に日夜響きます。爆心のこの地もまた水俣病なのです。

かつて、水俣湾は海の宝庫でした。回遊する魚たちは群れをなして産卵し、その稚魚たちはここで育ち成魚となり、また還ってくる母の胎のような所でした。百間から明神崎に至る現在の埋め立て地のあたりはイワシやコノシロが銀色のうろこを光らせボラが飛びかい、エビやカニがたわむれていました。潮のひいた海辺では貝を採り、波間に揺れるワカメやヒジキを採って暮らしてきました。私たちはこれらのいのちによって我が身を養う

Figure 7.1a "Hongan No Sho" or the Handwritten Mission Statement by Hongan No kai.

entails consuming other lives in order to maintain one's own life. Precisely because our lives are sustained at the expense of other lives, eating should not simply terminate lives but, rather, take other beings' "life-force" into one's own body. That act must be viewed not as mere consumption but as building a relationship; consuming and appreciating food, and thereby valuing lives, embodies the Hongan no kai's notion of the "vow for life." In this way, the term *hongan* does not indicate Buddhist salvation in a "pure land," but commitment to relations in this earthly realm (Figures 7.1a, b).

For Ogata and his fellow Hongan no kai members, Minamata disease not only caused the loss of their loved ones, of their own health, and of their livelihoods, but also shattered all relationships with their surroundings. These shattered relationships included familial bonds, community relations, and ties to the fish and shellfish of the sea—all of which sustained their living world. It is in the interest of rearticulating such relations that I have used Bennett's concept of "the agency of assemblages." However, the language of Hongan no kai members themselves would describe these relations using the religious terms *hongan* and *tamashii* that have been disregarded and marginalized in the modern secular world. More importantly, the members also aim to put into practice the commitments implied in their "vow." As we will now see, one such attempt by Hongan no kai involved carving stone statues and placing them on the reclaimed land of Minamata.

JIZŌ STATUES AND ECO PARK

Reflecting on the vow of Hongan no kai, Ogata remarks, "I think that Hongan no kai is a group dedicated to expressing itself in actions, in order to remember Minamata as well as to pray for all lives."[24] Hongan no kai, since its inception, has engaged in a praxis uniting members' ideas and actions. Accordingly, at its inauguration, Hongan no kai decided to carve stone statues of Jizō bodhisattva (Sanskrit: *Kṣitigarbha*) to place on the reclaimed land as an embodiment of the members' prayers to tamashii. The stone statues are conventionally called *Jizō* or *nobotoke* (Buddhist statue in the field). The latter term signifies that these figures are often found not on temple grounds but, rather, in fields (*no*). This spatial distance from institutional sites corresponds to and expresses the group's distance from official religious affiliation and authority.

Hongan no kai members also referred to the figures *tamashii ishi* (spirit stones). The members decided to place these figures on the 100 acres of reclaimed and beautified land in Minamata, discussed above. Upon

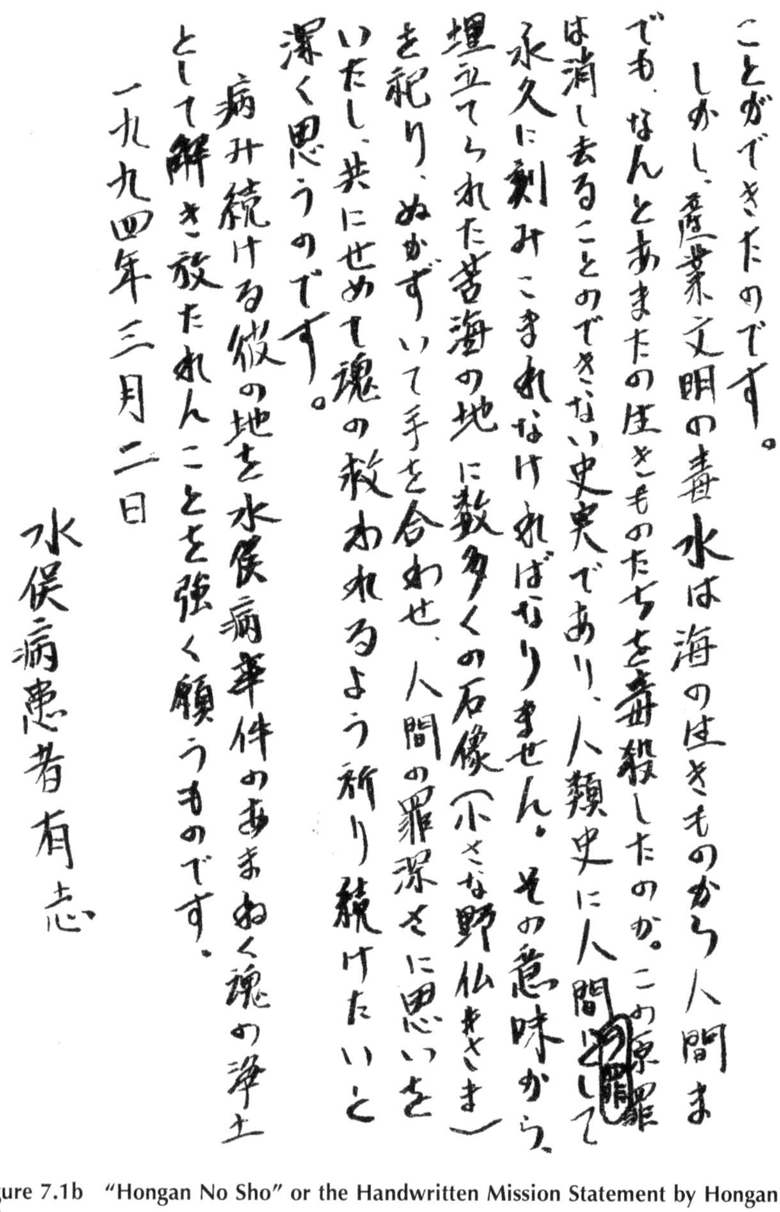
ことができたのです。
しかし、産業文明の毒水は海の生きものから人間までも、なんとあまたの生きものたちを毒殺したのか。この原罪は消し去ることのできない史実であり、人類史に人間の罪として永久に刻みこまれなければなりません。その意味から、埋立てられた苦海の地に数多くの石像（小さな野仏さま）を祀り、ぬかずいて手を合わせ、人間の罪深さに思いをいたし、共にせめて魂の救われるよう祈り続けたいと深く思うのです。
病み続ける彼の地を水俣病事件のあまねく魂の浄土として解き放たれんことを強く願うものです。
一九九四年三月二日
水俣病患者有志

Figure 7.1b "Hongan No Sho" or the Handwritten Mission Statement by Hongan No kai.

completion of the restoration, this site was rechristened as Eco Park—with athletic fields, a golf course, bamboo groves, rose gardens, and a scenic breakwater overlooking the Shiranui Sea.[25] On a small hill at the southwest tip of this reclaimed land, Minamatabyō shiryōkan (the Minamata Disease Municipal Museum), was erected with the purpose of informing the public about Minamata disease and its history. A manicured park with blooming flowers, growing trees, and lush shrubberies obscures the fact that this land is also a massive graveyard contaminated with methylmercury, in which countless dead fish, seashells, and other beings are buried.

To Hongan no kai members' minds, the reclaimed land should be a place in which visitors are invited to ponder Minamata disease and the sufferers' lives. They believe the knowledge about Minamata that visitors acquire at the museum should translate into actions that contemplate suffering and commemorate the dead. Upon the completion of Eco Park, Minamata City permitted Hongan no kai to take responsibility for an elongated strip of land in Eco Park facing the sea. The group chose to cultivate indigenous plants in this land with no need of artificial fertilizers, a gesture of ecological sustainability. They additionally decided to continue carving tamashii ishi, conducting rituals and offering prayers to invite spirits to enter the statues as they were placed on this site.[26]

However, once tamashii ishi were carved, Minamata City, the park's administrator, forbid the group from placing those stone statues on the land. This proscription was not issued because the city wished to suppress Hongan no kai's message, but rather because the city—as a secular governmental agency—could not allow any religious symbols in a public space.[27] In response to the city's rejection of the statues, Hongan no kai explained its rationale for carving and placing them in Eco Park. Ishimure, for example, wrote that the purpose of the statues was not to promulgate a religious doctrine but "to leave the footsteps of our lives."[28] Hamamoto Tsuginori, a founding member of Hongan no kai and a Minamata sufferer, expressed that the statues were for conveying to park visitors the suffering that resulted from Minamata disease and, in turn, for visitors to contemplate the plight of all beings—something he believed the municipal museum was ill equipped to do.[29]

Negotiating with the city for approval to continue placing statues in Eco Park, Hongan no kai members repeatedly explained that their actions were not religious in the sense of that term as commonly used in "secular" society; their actions did not aim to promote a religious institutional doctrine. Once the administration understood that Hongan no kai was unaffiliated with any religious institution and that their intention was not to evangelize a particular religious teaching, the city finally granted the group permission to place the tamashii ishi in Eco Park.[30]

Upon learning of Hongan no kai's practice of carving stone statues, Tanoue Yoshiharu—who had once served as the chair of Minamatabyō gojokai (Minamata Disease Mutual Aid Society) and Minamatabyō hoshō Tokyo kōshōdan (Minamata Disease Compensation Tokyo Negotiation Group)—was immediately convinced that carving these statues would now become his life's work. "Yes," he said, carving statues is "all we can do" to convey our vision. "We won't live long, we are not healthy."[31] Tanoue continued with

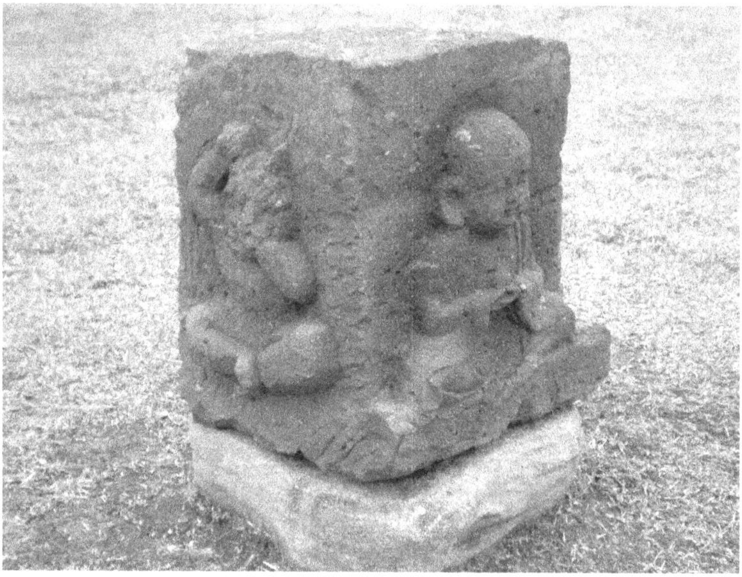

Figure 7.2 A Stone Statue in Eco Park Minamata. *Source:* Photo taken by the author.

laughter, "This is [Sugimoto] Eiko's idea, isn't it? It is religious or otherworldly. Ha-ha!"[32] Not conforming to particular religious traditions, Hongan no kai's tamashii ishi serve as a marker of the plight of all beings as well as a political statement—a means of communicating with the tamashii that were excluded from the museum's secular displays (Figures 7.2 and 7.3).

Over time, the statues have come to number over fifty. Although the bodhisattva Jizō remains the most prevalent carved figure, others have joined it. One now finds statues of Ebisu (the deity of fishers), Daruma (Bodhidharma), the Virgin Mary, a cat,[33] and even a Totoro lookalike (a popular character from the animated film *Tonari no Totoro*, or *My Neighbor Totoro*, released in 1988 by acclaimed animation director Miyazaki Hayao). These figures are so many avatars of the tamashii of the departed. A wide variety of figures thus stand on the reclaimed land at Eco Park, but it is worth inquiring into why the majority of the statues take the shape of Jizō—or at least why Hongan no kai members initially made Jizō figures.

Scholar of medieval Japanese religions Hank Glassman traces the history and popularity of Jizō. His monograph *The Face of Jizō: Image and Cult in Medieval Japanese Buddhism* explains particular attributes of Jizō in the minds of the Japanese people, illuminating the appeal of this figure to Hongan no kai members. Jizō is the name of a bodhisattva, but as Glassman observes, "Jizō" is also roughly used to signify any stone statue: "Old worn sculptural works in stone—statues or graves—all become 'Jizō,'"[34] he writes,

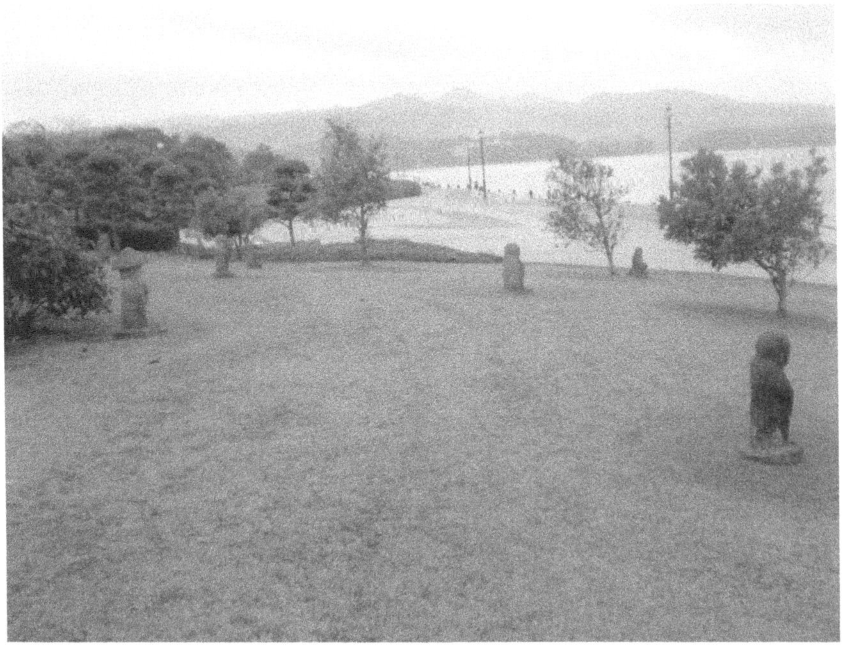

Figure 7.3 A Stone Statue in Eco Park Minamata. *Source:* Photo taken by the author.

thus including unidentified and deserted statues. Originally, Jizō bodhisattva was often depicted as an attendant to Buddha, assigned the task of serving as an intermediary between people and Buddha. Jizō's status as a bodhisattva, not yet an enlightened Buddha, makes Jizō rather more approachable to laypeople.

Yet Jizō's ambiguity—not yet enlightened but nonetheless an object of worship—also accounts for this rather peripheral status in the Buddhist hierarchy. Folklore scholar Gorai Shigeru points out that many temples place a statue of Amida Buddha in their main worship hall while placing a Jizō statue immediately outside their temple gates. The differences in these locations, Gorai asserts, corresponds to the hierarchical relationship between Amida and Jizō in Buddhist cosmology.[35] The location does not, however, mean that Jizō is excluded—rather, this location on the threshold of the temple signals Jizō's role as a guardian of borders. Tanoue explains Jizō's familiarity in everyday life, beyond institutional boundaries, in a manner that corresponds to Glassman's observations: "One finds Jizō statues not just in our neighborhood temples but all over Japan. Both elders and children put their hands together when they walk by a Jizō—our long-practiced custom."[36] The presence of Jizō's as a familiar figure that also resides just outside the borders of religious sites also speaks to its role in Eco Park, where it serves as a mediator between visitors to the park and Minamata sufferers.

Jizō's association with margins, borders, and in-between spaces may have been a transfer from the folkloric deity Dōsojin (Dōsoshin), or Sai no Kami—the deity who provides safe passage through the liminal space between villages. This folkloric figure's role is eventually taken on by the Buddhist figure of Jizō, who becomes a mediator between two realms, and is thus understood as a guardian for intersections and borders. In turn, Jizō comes to embody a compassionate companion on journeys. While Jizō is associated with intermediacy, liminality, and versatility, it is this aspect of companionship that accounts for Jizō's tenacious popularity. Glassman offers a Buddhist context for the emergence of this aspect: "Initial interest in Jizō in Japan begins from his role as an intercessor for the dead undergoing judgment and punishment in the infernal regions."[37] Over time, Jizō is imagined as a companion for the deceased on their journey to the underworld.

Companionship in times of transition is not limited to the end of life, but extends to the beginning as well. In premodern Japanese society, when newborns' mortality rate was high, children under six years of age were regarded as not yet fully human beings, but as still in the process of becoming human, making them liminal figures. Children were indeed regarded as belonging both to this earthly world and a world beyond. Jizō was considered a guardian figure for children, still in this transient phase of becoming fully fledged human beings. The close relationship between Jizō and children is evoked in figures of the deity, often represented with childlike traits, such as a round face. Jizō's adherents, meanwhile, don red bibs, much as children wear.[38] Because of this association between Jizō and children, some Hongan no kai members hope the Jizō statues will attract children. Other sufferers identify themselves with Jizō in his resemblance to children.

Jizō's role as mediator between worlds—and as a protector of liminal figures like children—eventually led women to rely on his power, particularly upon losing a child to miscarriage, illness, accident, or abortion.[39] Believing that Jizō would assist a child's smooth transition from this world to the world beyond, mothers and caregivers of lost children often found comfort in his image. The Jizō statues placed in Minamata represent children as well. As Ishimure attests, "One excruciating fact about Minamata disease was to see the suffering of babies and children. Some women lost their babies, and others gave birth to babies with congenital problems. The countless number of miscarriage cases was unrecorded. . . . If the stone statues [in Eco Park] remind visitors of those lost lives, they may stop their walks to consider the meaning of the statues."[40]

Beyond its affiliation with thresholds, passages, and liminal spaces and beings, the Jizō figure carries cultural, historical, and religious meanings that extends to its very materiality. Hongan no kai's choice of stone, rather than wood, for the statues was carefully considered. As Ishimure notes, Japanese folklore suggests that stone, like wood, contains tamashii. Petrologist Yoshikawa Muneaki notes that stones have been an objects of worship in Japan, which were adopted in Shinto and Buddhism.[41] Hongan no kai's choice of stone personally pleased Ishimure because her father and grandfather had been masons. Recalling a childhood memory, Ishimure writes about their masonry work, which included carving the Yakushi Nyorai (Bhaisajyaguru), or Medicine Buddha,[42] and stone guardian dog statues for a Shinto shrine. In addition, they collected stones and with them built walls, laid foundations for roads and bridges, erected tombstones, and constructed memorials.[43] Thanks to her family's business, Ishimure grew up believing that one of the greatest figures in this world is a deity called "Seishoko sama." At the time she had no knowledge of this deity beyond its name, but later Ishimure would learn that *Seishoko* referred to a historical figure and local Kumamoto lord, Katō Kiyomasa (1562–1611). Since the name Kiyomasa can also be read in Chinese characters as *seishō*, *Lord Seishō* (*Seishō kō*) eventually became *Seishoko* among the commoners.[44] The suffix "*sama*" is an honorific, thus Seishokosama means the *Honorable Lord Shishō*.

Kumamoto is known for the great skill of its masons. Kumamoto Castle, for example—built by Kiyomasa or Seishō kō—is particularly distinguished for its sturdy stone construction. Ishimure informs her readers that even the large-scale earthquake that hit Kumamoto City in 2016 did not completely destroy the stone walls of the castle's foundation. The parts that survived had been erected in Kiyomasa's time, while those that collapsed were a later addition. Ishimure fondly remembers that her father would say, with ingenuous awe evident on his face, "I would not be able to face Seishoko sama if I prioritized money in accepting job offers."[45] Thus, the stone deity, associated with an actual historical figure, held a special place among the masons in Kumamoto. Ishimure thus found spiritual significance in the fact that she—the daughter of a mason from the Shiraishi household,[46] whose name carries the Chinese characters for "stone" (*ishi*)—married a man whose last name, Ishimure, also contains "stone" (*ishi*).

On nights before placing a stone statue on the reclaimed land, Hongan no kai members and supporters hold a gathering, called a *goya*, to pray together.[47] They enact this ritual in order to invite a spirit to enter the statue. When unable to hold a *goya*, they instead offer saké to the new statue on the day of its placement.[48] Kanazashi notes that it was Ishimura who initially proposed these gatherings in front of the statues. At the time, Ishimure further suggested bringing lanterns to the site, borrowing this idea from a local *Hi no matsuri*, or fire festival. To make the lantern fire more visible, the better to guide the spirits, Hongan no kai members and supporters thus decided to bring torches instead of lanterns to conduct the first goya. Unfortunately, due to a Minamata City regulation forbidding the display of fire in public spaces, they had to give up the torches. They therefore began to hold the goya gatherings, without torches, before each new stone statue.[49]

As Hongan no kai, along with supporters, added more statues to the reclaimed land, Minamata City inquired with Hongan no kai about the number of statues they planned to place. Kanazashi responded, "We do not plan ahead. We would like to continue to place the statues as long as possible."[50] Since the Jizō statues are the medium connecting visitors to Eco Park and tamashii, the group continues to carve a new statue whenever they feel that one is necessary, following intuitions that can neither be planned nor administrated. The city's inquiry concerning Hongan no kai's intention to continue making statues highlights different attitudes toward memorials: for the city, considering the number of statues that can go into a limited space was rational thinking, but for Hongan no kai, the frequency with which one should remember the dead and communicate with tamashii is simply not a matter of calculation.

Thus, carving the statues and placing them in Eco Park is both a salient political and spiritual gesture for Hongan no kai. Resisting the secular municipal museum's attempt to domesticate the sufferer's history by withholding space for open-ended communication with tamashii, Hongan no kai seeks to supplement the city's narrative *indefinitely* with their ongoing placement of Jizō statues. By carving and placing these statues, they invite visitors to consider the suffering of all beings, to communicate with tamashii, and to envision a world that operates very differently, with an ontology and epistemology distinct from that of this secular world. Hongan no kai's praxis intervenes into and gently disrupts the municipally managed park, giving the group and all who care to do so a place in which to communicate with tamashii. This dissonance brings visitors to a halt and instigates questions that invite contemplation: What are these figures? Why are they here? What are they for?

THIS WORLD AND A WORLD OTHERWISE

Thus far, I have described Hongan no kai's attempts to demonstrate and realize members' vision of a world otherwise through prayers, rituals, literature, and stone carvings. But Hongan no kai does not intend to displace or to replace this world with the group's vision of a world otherwise. This kind of transformation *must* happen, and yet it *cannot be coerced*. Ogata states, "One should not identify *sukui* (salvation or relief) with social change. . . . When we aim at social change, we try to control others."[51] For Ogata, the way to change is not by dominating the world with his vision, but by seeking to realize a world otherwise in its openness and multiplicity.

Given this context, some of Ogata's more enigmatic statements may be rendered more comprehensible. Ogata often emphasizes his resistance to becoming part of this world's majority, commenting, "Inviting people to our events is not a means for us to become the majority [of this world]. On the contrary, if we become the majority, that would be counted as a failure." Within the overbearingly enlarged system of this world—the world of predatory corporations, municipal administrations, nationalistic aspirations—"I am merely passing time."[52] For Ogata, becoming the majority would mean participating in the "overbearing system" and conforming to its rules and structures—the very things that lead to oppression and suffering. Ogata's world otherwise is a world both within and against the modern world, the world of the "majority."

Though Ogata wishes to avoid identifying salvation with social change, moving between the two worlds—this world and a world otherwise—is not a disengagement from ethical responsibility. To live in at least these two realms means, for Ogata, to be accountable for both worlds. In more concrete terms, he analogizes the modern ostensibly secular world with Japan, and a world otherwise with *shōgoku,* or "birthplace." The former indicates the realm of a sovereign political entity whose laws, regulations, and norms we inevitably, if sometimes partially, abide, whether consciously or not. The latter does not necessarily suggest a physical birthplace; it may be a real, geographically identifiable place, or a mythic realm, much like Ishimure's understanding of furusato.

In Ogata's personal cosmology, shōgoku is the Shiranui Sea—the waters next to which he was born, by which he was nurtured, and to which he will eventually return. For other people, shōgoku can be an actual birthplace, visible on a map, or an invisible, imaginary space. Ogata considers *shōgoku* to be a place in which one's life, and indeed all lives, are treated as precious elements of an intimately interconnected world. As Ogata's example makes clear, to live genuinely in shōgoku—to *realize* shōgoku—is the opposite of escapism, for it entails living in recognition of the agency of assemblages, and thus to act with care in accepting one's influence over other beings and, at the same time, others' influence over one's own existence. This means valuing, in one's actions and attitude toward the world, the lives of all and, in turn, discerning and responding to the precarity that characterizes the modern world. As we have already seen in the discourse of furusato, the modern world, so often characterized by anthropocentrism, profit margins, and nationalist sentiment, might demand self-sacrifice on the part of its subjects, coerced by the moral rhetoric of *loyalty* and *courage*. But living in multiple worlds—a world otherwise that is at once within and against the modern world—offers a perspective that allows us better to discern whose interests are served, and at whose expense those interests come, under the social norms that reproduce precarity. Too often, moral codes serve to maintain and reinforce the structures that benefit a privileged few while rendering the lives of others precarious.

For this reason, Ogata suggests "futatsu no kuni o ikiru," or having "dual citizenship" in this world and in the shōgoku.[53] In Sōshisha's 2006 newsletter, *Gonzui*, Ogata expounds upon his notion of residing in two worlds. "In the Edo period [1604–1868]," Ogata comments,

> there is the shogunate and its authority. Under this oppressive power structure, people still had to seek a way to live their own lives and to survive in their own community. We need to regain the wisdom of living skillfully between two worlds—that of the state and that of one's community. At present, one has to offer one's obedience to authority by observing rules and regulations made in Tokyo, but one simultaneously should pursue one's own way of life, not necessarily conforming to the norms promoted by governmental authority.[54]

Traveling between the two worlds—that is, between a world organized and managed by a centralized political authority (whether in the form of the shogunate or the modern nation-state) and one's shōgoku (whether in the form of one's immediate community or an imagined "birthplace")—requires the wherewithal to dwell in ambiguity, in the multiple values of a world of assemblages and "vital, crosscutting forces."[55] Indeed, Hongan no kai members find the ability to travel between the two worlds crucial. I see this ability as a new ethical element.

Ogata's dual citizenship is not, therefore, a matter of duplicity, but rather an expression of prudence and sagacity—an approach that relies not, or not exclusively, on external authority but, as Hongan no kai members have demonstrated, on the wisdom of accumulated personal experience and one's shōgoku.[56] Yet, this kind of dual citizenship may be dismissed or looked down on as irrational according to the implicit understanding of rationality in "secular" society. But Ishimure shares with Mahmood a suspicion of the supposed rationality of secular society itself. Recognizing that "modernity" claims to "[value] rationality" despite the acts of discrimination, exploitation, and violence perpetrated under its guise, Ishimure asks, "What is rationality?"[57] "Calculating thoroughly so that one will avoid any monetary loss?" Secular modernity advocates calculative logic in the service of profit and power, mandating acts that are, to her mind, unethical and irrational. Recalling the measures that "rational" individuals and institutions will take in the interest of accruing profit and eschewing penalty, Ishimure concludes that "the purpose of modernity is to enable the collective to execute the destruction of evidence and the shirking of responsibility [without legal penalty]."[58]

Ishimure thus contends that the moral claim to rationality is too often nothing more than part of a self-serving rhetoric legitimating acts of self-interest to the detriment of already precarious lives. In short, the moral claims of rationality are undermined by the immoral acts, while the rhetoric of rationality is used to justify such acts.

Echoing Ishimure, William Rasch cites legal scholar Martti Koskenniemi's term *rational imperialism*[59] in criticizing what we perceive as "rational."[60] According to Rasch and Koskenniemi, what constitutes *rationality* stands on no logical ground and is only tautological—that is, what many people *perceive* as rational *is* rational. Or, as Rasch explains, "There is no universal mode of legitimation [of reason] that could adjudicate the dispute between reason and what the reasonable define as *nonreason*."[61] If Ishimure and Rasch are right, what we call "rationality" only points to the thoughts and behaviors that serve to sustain the ideologies underwriting current political and economic systems, supporting the individuals who benefit from those systems and disadvantaging others.

In this world where nearly everything may be commodified, used, and valued according to the dictates of the market, resisting a "rational" modality entails creating and embracing values that undermine the foundation of this secular modern world. Philosopher Slavoj Žižek's discussion of ecology, for example, aligns with Hongan no kai's attempts to question what constitutes rationality as well as the group's advocacy for an ontological and epistemological shift to a world otherwise. "The conservative critics of modernity," writes Žižek, "claim we should not get too involved with technology. Instead, we should rediscover simple pleasures of walking in the forest, sitting at a table, just drinking water, whatever, that is still part of a technological universe for me."[62] Occasional camping trips and outings in "nature" do not produce ecological change or reverse environmental crises; still worse, such activities often amount to further exploitation or "use" of nature for recreational pleasure, observes Žižek. He goes on to discuss the need for emotional investment and genuine interaction with our surroundings, going beyond the logic of utility, claiming that a "true spiritual change [must] develop . . . a kind of emotional attachment to, or . . . find meaning in, useless objects."[63]

"Emotional attachment" that finds "meaning in useless objects" contributes to the cultivation of an attitude of valuation not restricted to use value or dictated by the market. And this idea of emotional investment in that which exceeds utility—that which appears irrational from the "secular rationalist" perspective, but actually reveals the illogic and violence of the "rational" secular world—has been repeatedly demonstrated by Hongan no kai's members. Sugimoto Eiko's notion of nosari, Ishimure Michiko's mythopoetic furusato, Ogata Masato's shōgoku, and Hongan no kai's tamashii ishi: each of these is a starting point, a creative implement for envisioning and *realizing* our own worlds otherwise. Claiming dual citizenship between the modern world and a world otherwise means perceiving the value of that which modern secular society deems "useless"—including those who are marginalized by illness, displaced by environmental catastrophe, or whose lives are made precarious under the dictates of nation and market.

The planned shukkongi for the 1996 Minamata exhibition, which I discussed at the beginning of this chapter, had a sequel. Ogata's wooden boat, the Nichigetsumaru, reached Tokyo safely and was exhibited onsite. On October 16, 1996, after closing the exhibition, Hongan no kai members and their supporters held a *tamashii gaeshi no gi* (a ritual of returning tamashii) in Shinagawa, Tokyo, during which the Nichigetsumaru was disassembled. At this ritual, participants offered flowers to the boat as a token of gratitude, and the vessel was ultimately cremated.[64] Afterward, 200 tons of metal were recycled and made into a miniature Nichigetsumaru, one-seventh of the actual size, which was exhibited at Minamata City's Moyai Naoshi Center.[65]

Four years later, on August 13, 2000, Hongan no kai gathered near the bamboo woods at Eco Park, where they held another shukkongi to reunite with tamashii of the Minamata sufferers, both human and nonhuman.[66] In the middle of a grassy space, they prepared an altar on which they offered saké, *shōchū* (a distilled alcohol), salt, rice, seven herbs of autumn (*aki no nanakusa*), rice cakes, rice balls, fried chicken, fish paste cakes, fish, seaweeds, vegetables, and so on. Beside the altar platform, participants placed paper lanterns made of Kanazashi's special washi. Candles emitted warm, gentle light, and incense gave off a soothing fragrance. Across the altar hung the banner of the Nichigetsumaru.[67] The ritual began with a performance by members of "Take no honoo" (bamboo flame), local youths playing musical instruments made of bamboo. Then Sugimoto Eiko walked to the altar and clasped her hands in prayer, in which the audience joined.[68] Finally, the ashes of the Nichigetsumaru were placed in an urn and buried between the two tamashii ishi, carved by Sugimoto Takeshi and Ishimure Hiroshi, bearing Jizō's likeness.

Hongan no kai's practice has thus demonstrated the agency of assemblages in creatively communicating with tamashii through their rituals. Hagihara Shūko, a scholar of religion who examines the ethical responses of Minamata disease sufferers, explains that Hongan no kai "does not have a consensus on the definitions of such common terms as 'spirit,' 'life,' or 'prayer,' but, on the contrary, each member continues to ask ceaselessly what these words mean to her."[69] The group's conscious refusal to fix definitions is a unique facet of its members' willingness to self-reflection and openness to multivalent, ambiguous worlds. Indeed, ambiguity and openness may be crucial to the kind of critical self-reflection that Hongan no kai sees as essential for claiming dual citizenship. "The Minamata disease incident manifests how terribly our modern industrialized society is suffering. We must not forget that underneath the incident is our own sin and arrogance, which led us to the destruction of our environment and of the invaluable lives of people."[70]

Living out their alternative ontology, Hongan no kai has transformed the tip of Eco Park into a space where one may contemplate the tamashii of humans, nonhumans, and other-than humans. It is a place in which the sufferers of Minamata disease may speak their wisdom. This alternative space, like a Noh stage, thus facilitates communication with other-than-human existences, such as tamashii, genius loci, and the dead. I believe that in creating this space, Hongan no kai has also shown how members conceive of a true moyai naoshi, a binding-together—establishing relations with oneself and with others avoiding withdrawing into nostalgia. Reflecting the mission statement that was declared at its inception, Hongan no kai is able to conjure a world otherwise within—and against—the modern world that would seek to exclude it.

However, as we have seen, in our secular society, the language of tamashii, like other aspects of a world otherwise, may sound irrational or be met with aversion. But for Hongan no kai, this aversion itself evidences the efficacy of their religious language, rituals, and images, which quietly challenge the norms of a secular world whose violent "rationality" too often comports with harm. Abandoning both economic self-interest that destroys humans and the environment on the one hand and politically coerced self-sacrifice on the other, Hongan no kai encourages a spirit of self-*giving*—a form of nosari that, like the tamashii with which it assembles, may circulate in our midst, creating a more vital and intimately connected world.

NOTES

1. Yonemoto, Koji, *Hyouden Ishimure Michiko: Nagisa ni tatsu hito* (Critical biography of Ishimure Michiko: A Person Who Stands on the Beach) (Tokyo: Shinchōsha, 2017), 250.

2. Yonemoto, *Hyouden Ishimure Michiko*, 250. Ishimure says, "Putting together the sun (*niche*) and the moon *(getsu*), *Nichigetsumaru.* Without *nichigetsu,* the earth would not have existed."

3. Hongan no, kai, "Minamata chikurinen shukkongi" (Minamata bamboo garden shukkongi), *Tamashii utsure* 3 (2000): 2; Kakuta Toyoko, "Kosame no naka inochi matsuru gishiki" (A ritual to celebrate the life in the rain), *Tamashii utsure* 11 (2002): 4.

4. Ritsumeikan Daigaku Global COE Program, "'Seizongaku' souseikyoten, 'Rekishi no naka ni okeru toi: Kurihara Akira sensei ni kiku'" (Questions in history: interviewing professor Kurihara Akira). Ritsumeikan Daigaku Seizongaku

Kenkyu Center: 37, www.ritsumei-arsvi.org/publications/read/id/26; Junpei Kanazashi, "Watashi no Minamata" (My Minamata), *Tamashii utsure* 1 (1998): 25.

5. I follow the spelling for the Prophet's name that Saba Mahmood uses in the following essay: Mahmood, "Religious Reason and Secular Affect," 65.

6. Mahmood, "Religious Reason and Secular Affect," 83, 85.

7. Mahmood, "Religious Reason and Secular Affect," 83–88.

8. For example, Wendy Brown claims that the fact that major Christian holidays, including Sundays, conveniently fall on the weekend or during breaks is not a coincidence but, rather, proof that our society has religious underpinnings. See Wendy Brown, *Regulating Aversion: Tolerance in the Age of Identity and Empire* (Princeton; NJ: Princeton University Press, 2006), especially Chapter Seven: "Tolerance as/in Civilizational Discourse."

9. William Rasch, "Enlightenment as Religion," *New German Critique* 36, no. 3 (2009): 113–114.

10. Rasch, "Enlightenment as Religion," 113–115. For the discourse of tolerance, see Brown, *Regulating Aversion,* Chapter Seven.

11. Rasch, "Enlightenment as Religion," 116.

12. Indeed, the recent rightward trend has found support in Nippon Kaigi, an ultraconservative political group based upon Shinto ideology. See, for example, Aike P. Rots, "Sacred Forests, Sacred Nation: The Shinto Environmentalist Paradigm and the Rediscovery of *Chinju no Mori,*" *Japanese Journal of Religious Studies,* 42, no. 2 (2015): 205–233.

13. Ishimure, Michiko, "Tatoe hitori ni nattemo" (Even I was left alone), *Tamashii utsure,* 1 (1998): 2.

14. Tanno, Haruka, "Yanagida Kōichi to 'Minamatabyō o tsutaeru' katsudō': Shisui no kihon kōzō o chūshin ni" (Kōichi Yanagida and passing down activities on Minamata disease: focusing on the fundamental structure of his ideas), *Kankyō kyōiku* 25, no. 1 (2015): 50–51.

15. Tanno, "Yanagida Kōichi to 'Minamatabyō o tsutaeru' undō,'" 51.

16. Kanazashi, Junpei, "Omae wa nanimono da" (Who are you?), *Tamashii utsure* 5 (2001): 24.

17. Chisso paid 30,600,000,000 Japanese yen of the total cost of 48,500,000,000 yen.

18. Hongan no kai, "Zadankai: Inochi no negai o oimotomete" (Roundtable: searching for the lives' vow), *Tamashii utsure* 36 (2009): 9.

19. Hara, Takeshi, "Intabyū Ogata Masato: 'Bunmei no kakumei' o machinozomu—Hongan towa nani ka" (Interview Ogata Masato: waiting for the revolution of civilization—what is the original vow?), in *Kyoto Kankyōgaku: Shūkyōsei to ekorojī* (Kyoto environmental studies: Religiosity and ecology), ed. Hara Takeshi (Tokyo: Fujiwara shoten, 2013), 140.

20. Hara, "Intabyū Ogata Masato," 140

21. Hara, "Intabyū Ogata Masato," 143.

22. Shinshū Temple in Kumamoto City offered a workspace in 1987 to Ishimure Michiko, who was also drawn to Shinran's thoughts. Since then, this temple has become a hub in Kumamoto City for Hongan no kai.

23. Ogata, Masato, in *Tamashii utsure* (Transforming the spirit) 36 (2009): 7.
24. Ishimure, *Soseishita tamashii o nosete*, 191.
25. The official website of Minamata City: http://minamata-kouen.com/.
26. Yoshinaga, Rimiko, "Umetatechi no iwa ni horitai, 7-nen buri 'tamashii ishi (nobutsu)' hori saikai" (We want to carve the stone on the reclaimed land: resuming carving the *tamashii ishi*, or *nobutsu*, after seven years), *Tamashii utsure* 48 (2011): 24.
27. "Inochi no negai o oimotomete" (Roundtable: seeking for the wishes of lives), *Tamashii utsure* 36 (2009): 9. In this roundtable, Sugimoto Takashi said, "Especially Kumamoto prefecture strongly opposed."
28. Ishimure, "Tatoe hitori ni nattemo," 2.
29. Hamamoto, Tsuginori, "Goaisatsu" (Greetings), *Tamashii utsure* 1 (1998): i.
30. Kanazashi, Junpei, "'Hongan no kai' towa nani ka" (What is Hongan no kai?), *Tamashii utsure* 7 (2001): 4.
31. Ishimure, "Tatoe hitori ni nattemo," 3.
32. Ishimure, "Tatoe hitori ni nattemo," 3.
33. Kanazashi, "Watashi no Minamata," 26.
34. Hank Glassman, *The Face of Jizō: Image and Cult in Medieval Japanese Buddhism* (Honolulu, HI: University of Hawai'i Press, 2012), 188.
35. Gorai, Shigeru, *Ishi no shūkyō* (Religion of the stone) (Tokyo: Kadokawa shoten, 1988), 56.
36. Ishimure, *Sosei shita tamashii o nosete*, 27.
37. Glassman, *The Face of Jizō*, 15.
38. The color red is closely linked with celebration and considered transitory to the next life stage. A newborn baby is called *aka-chan*, meaning "a little red." Also, the custom of wearing a red vest upon reaching the age of sixty is still practiced, originating in times when reaching sixty was extraordinary.
39. See William R. LaFleur, *Liquid Life: Abortion and Buddhism in Japan* (Princeton: Princeton University Press, 1994). Also, Milla Micka Moro-Sanchez examines the healing and empowerment of women through rituals of Jizō worship in Japan. See Milla Micka Moro-Sanchez, "Jizō, Healing Rituals, and Women in Japan," *Japanese Journal of Religious Studies* 43, no. 2 (2016): 307–331.
40. Ishimure, *Sosei shita tamashii o nosete*, 79.
41. Yoshikawa, Muneaki, *Ganseki o shinkō shite ita Nihonjin: Ishigami, iwakura, iwasaka, kigan, kyoseki to yobareru mono no kenkyū* (Japanese who worshipped the stone: a study on the stone deity, the dwelling place of the stone deity, the territorial border of the stone deity, the strangely shaped stone, and the megalith) (Osaka: Yū taimu shuppan, 2011), 41.
42. Ishimure, Michiko, *Yoshi no nagisa* (On the beach of reed) (Tokyo: Fujiwara shoten, 2014), 237.
43. Ishimure, Michiko, *Tamashii no hikyō kara* (Untrodden corner of my spirit) (Tokyo: Asahi shimbunsha, 2018), 26.
44. The Chinese characters of Kiyomasa can be read as "Seishō." He was also known as Seishō *kō*, or Lord Seishō. *Seishoko*, in Ishimure's memory, derives from *Seishō kō*.

45. Ishimure, *Tamashii no hikyō kara,* 197.

46. Shiraishi is Ishimure's mother's maiden name.

47. *Goya* refers to a widely observed vigil in Kumamoto in which festival participants stayed up to protect the deities on the night before a festival.

48. Shimoda, Kentarō, "Minamatawan umetatechi no 52 tai no sekizō tachi, Jou: soko kara miete kurumono" (Fifty-two stone statues on the reclaimed land of Minamata, part 1: what is seen from there), *Tamashii utsure* 51 (2012): 27.

49. Kanazashi, Junpei, "Inochi no negai o oimotomete" (Hongan no kai roundtable: pursuing the wish of lives), *Tamashii utsure* 36 (2009): 11.

50. Kanazashi, "'Hongan no kai' towa nani ka," 4.

51. Ogata, "Tokoyo no fune o kogite," 188.

52. Ogata, "Tokoyo no fune o kogite," 188.

53. Ogata, Masato, "Kichō kōen 'Souseiki o mukaeta Minamata'" (Keynote speech: "Minamata at the dawn of new era"), *Tamashii utsure* 29 (2007): 5–6. For Ogata's translation of *moyai,* see Chapter 3, note 61.

54. Ogata, Masato, "Hontou no 'kuni' o motomete" (Seeking the true "nation"), *Gonzui* 95 (2006): 94.

55. Bennett, *Vibrant Matter*, 38.

56. Perhaps Ogata's suggestion about the sagacity of living in two realms might be understood a *hōben.* The distinction between *deception* and *expedience* may resonate with, and better explained by, the Buddhist term *hōben* (*upaya* in Sanskrit; *fāngbiàn* in Chinese), conventionally translated as "expediency," "skillful means," or "adapted teachings." See Daigan Matsunaga and Alicia Matsunaga, "The Concept of Upāya in Mahāyāna Buddhist Philosophy," *Japanese Journal of Religious Studies,* 1, no. 1 (1974): 51. The Mahāyāna tradition holds that Buddha's vast and profound teachings must be taught according to students' ability to learn. A Buddhist text, the *Lotus Sutra* (Sadharmapundarīka), gives the example of hōben being taught through a parable about a burning house. Children were playing inside a house when the house caught fire. The father outside urged them to come out of the house, but the children, not noticing the fire, refused to do so since they were enjoying playing in the house. The father made several attempts to no avail. Finally, the father called out to the children, "If you come out now, you can play with new and better toys!" Upon hearing these words, the children ran out of the house in excitement and saved themselves from the fire. This strategy that saved the children's lives is *hōben,* and the text explains, "It is the working of the mysterious, the excellent, *upāya.*" See Alan L. Miller, "Spiritual Accomplishment by Misdirection: Some 'Upāya' Folktales from East Asia," *History of Religions,* 40, no. 1 (2000): 83.

57. "Ishimure Michiko san ni kiku 'Watashi ni totte Chisso towa nani de attanoka'" (Interviewing Ishimure Michiko: "What Was Chisso for Her?"), *Tamashii utsure,* 41 (2010): 13.

58. "Ishimure Michiko san ni kiku 'Watashi ni totte Chisso towa nani de attanok,'" 13.

59. Martti Koskenniemi, *The Gentle Civilizer of Nations: The Rise and Fall of International Law 1870–1960* (New York: Cambridge University Press, 2001), 491.

60. Rasch, "Enlightenment as Religion," 109–131.

61. Rasch, "Enlightenment as Religion," 123.

62. Slavoj Žižek, "Ecology," in *Examined Life: Excursions with Contemporary Thinkers,* ed. Astra Taylor (New York: The New Press, 2009), 164.

63. Žižek, "Ecology,"163.

64. Mukai, Miwako, "Watashi no yamai toshite tsugi no sedai ni" (My illness to the next generation), *Tamashii utsure* 1 (1998): 21.

65. Hongan no kai, *Tamashii utsure* 4 (2001): 30.

66. Hongan no kai, "Minamata Chikurin'en Shukkongi" (Shukkongi at Minamata bamboo woods), *Tamashii utsure* 3 (2000): 2.

67. Tsunoda, Toyoko, "Kosame no naka inochi matsuru gishiki" (A ritual to celebrate the life in a shower), *Tamashii utsure* 11 (2002): 4.

68. Tsunoda, "Kosame no naka inochi matsuru gishiki," 5.

69. Hagihara, Shūko, "Umiotosareru kotoba, tewatasareteiku kotoba: Minamatabyō jiken to 'Hongan no kai.'" (Words brought forth, words handed down: The Minamata disease incident and 'Hongan no kai'), *Shūkyō kenkyū* 373 (2011), 209.

70. *Tamashii utsure* 1 (1998). The English translation was original. In this document, *Tamashii utsure* 6 (2001): 5, they call themselves "Club of the Original Vow," but I will provide their Japanese name, Hongan no kai, throughout this book.

References

COMPILED DOCUMENTS

Minamatabyō jishu kōshō Kawamoto saiban shiryōshū. 1981.
Minamatabyō jiken shiryōshū. 1996.

NEWSPAPERS, NEWSLETTERS

Asahi shimbun
Gaia Minamata
Gonzui
Japan Times
Kumamoto Nichinichi shimbun
Mainichi shimbun
Minamata kōjō shimbun
Reuters
Shin Nihon Chisso rōdō kumiai kikanshi, Sairen.
Tamashii utsure

FILMS AND TV PROGRAMS

Charles, Larry. 2008. *Religulous.*
NHK, *Nihonjin wan ani o mezashite kitanka Chi no kyojin tachi,* vol. 6, *Kindai towa nanika, Tamashii no yukue, Sakka Ishimure Michiko.* January 17, 2015.
Tsuchimoto, Noriaki. 1971. *Minamata: The Victims and Their World.*

WEBSITES

Fukushima Prefectural website
Minamata City website

SECONDARY SOURCES

Adelstein, Jake and David McNeill. "Meltdown: What Really Happened at Fukushima?" *The Atlantic,* July 2, 2017. https://www.theatlantic.com/international/archive/2011/07/meltdown-what-really-happened-fukushima/352434/.

Agamben, George. *Remnants of Auschwitz: The Witness and the Archive,* trans. by Daniel Hellier-Roazen. New York: Zone Books, 2002.

Allen, Bruce. "Facing the True Costs of Living." In *Coming into Contact: Explorations in Ecocritical Theory and Practice,* edited by Annie Merrill Ingram, Ian Marshall, Daniel J. Philippon, and Adam W Sweeting, 154–67. Athens, GA: University of Georgia Press, 2007.

_______. "Introduction" to Ishimure Michiko's *Lake of Heaven.* Translated by Bruce Allen. Lanham, MD: Rowman & Littlefield, 2008.

_______. "Secret Song." *World Literature Today* 82, no. 4 (2008): 31–35.

_______. "The Noh Imagination in Shiranui and the Work of Ishimure Michiko." In *Ishimure Michiko's Writing in Ecocritical Perspective: Between Sea and Sky,* edited by Bruce Allen and Yuki Masami, 173–188. Lanham, MD: Lexington Books, 2016.

Ambros, Barbara R. "Partaking of Life: Buddhism, Meat-Eating, and Sacrificial Discourses of Gratitude in Contemporary Japan." *Religions* 10, no. 4 (2019), https://www.mdpi.com/2077-1444/10/4/279#cite.

Amino, Yoshihiko. *Kaimin to Nihonshakai.* Tokyo: Sin jinbutsu oraisha, 2009 [1998].

_______. *Umi no kuni no chūsei.* Tokyo: Heibonsha, 1997.

Aoyama, Kōji. *Tatakai no kouzu,* vols. 1 and 2. Tokyo: Asahi shimbunsha, 1991.

Apffel-Marglin, Frédérique. *Subversive Spiritualities: How Rituals Enact the World.* New York: Oxford University Press, 2011.

Asad, Ralal. *Genealogies of Religion: Discipline and Reasons of Power in Christianity and Islam.* Baltimore, MD: Johns Hopkins University Press, 2013.

Bauman, Zygmunt. *Liquid Modernity.* Cambridge: Polity, 2000.

Beck, Ulrich. *Risk Society: Towards a New Modernity.* New York: Sage Publications, 1992.

_______. *World Risk Society.* Cambridge: Polity, 1999.

Bennett, Jane. *The Enchantment of Modern Life: Attachments, Crossings, and Ethics.* Princeton: Princeton University Press, 2001.

_______. *Vibrant Matter: A Political Ecology of Things.* Durham, NC: Duke University Press, 2010.

Berger, John. *G.* New York: Vintage Books, 1972.

Boyer, Dominic. "Anthropology Electric." *Cultural Anthropology* 30, no. 4. (2015): 531–39.

Brown, Wendy. *Regulating Aversion: Tolerance in the Age of Identity and Empire.* Princeton: Princeton University Press, 2006.
Butler, Judith. *Precarious Life: The Powers of Mourning and Violence.* London: Verso, 2004.
_______. *Frames of War: When Is Life Grievable?* London: Verso, 2009.
Butler, Judith and Athanasiou, Atena. *The Performative in the Political.* Malden, MA: Polity, 2013.
Camus, Albert. *Neither Victims nor Executioners: An Ethic Superior to Murder.* Translated by Dwight Macdonald. Eugene, OR: Wipf & Stock, 1946 [1986].
Cavanaugh, William T. *The Myth of Religious Violence.* New York: Oxford University Press, 2009.
Ding, Weiwei. "Fukushima genpatsu jiko to 'Minamata' gensetsu ni kansuru ichikousatsu: Kanrenshiryou no bunseki o rei ni." *Mediagaku: Bunka to komyunikēshon,* 29 (2014): 85–97.
Eckert, Carter J. *Offspring of Empire: The Koch'ang Kims and the Colonial Origins of Korean Capitalism, 1876–1945.* Seattle, WA: University of Washington Press 2014.
Field, Norma. "'Heiwa to han'ei' no ato de: Shikago daigaku meiyo kyoju Norma Field-san ni kiku." *Asahi Shimbun,* March 1, 2014.
_______. "This Will Still Be True Tomorrow: 'Fukushima Ain't Got the Time for Olympic Games': Two Texts on Nuclear Disaster and Pandemic." *The Asia-Pacific Journal,* 18, issue 13, no. 2 (2020), https://apjjf.org/2020/13/MutoField.html
Foucault, Michel. *Discipline and Punish: The Birth of the Prison.* Translated by Alan Sheridan. New York: Vintage Books, 1977.
Fujiwara, Shin'ya. *Yomi no inu.* Tokyo: Bungei shunjū, 2006.
Fukai, Jun'ichi. *Minamatabyō no seijikeizaigaku: Sangyōshiteki haikei to gyousei sekinin.* Tokyo: Keisō shobō, 1999.
Gaulène, Mathieu. "Does the Advertising Giant Dentsu Pull the Strings of the Japanese Media?" Translated by Sachie Mizohata. *The Asia-Pacific Journal* 14, issue 11, no. 5 (2016), https://apjjf.org/2016/11/Gaulene.html
George, Timothy S. *Minamata: Pollution and the Struggle for Democracy in Postwar Japan.* Cambridge, MA: Harvard University Asia Center, 2001.
Giddens, Anthony. *Modernity and Self-Identity: Self and Society in the Late Modern Age.* Stanford: Stanford University Press, 1991.
Ginoza, Naomi. *Modan raifu to sensou—sukurīn no naka no joseitachi.* Tokyo: Yoshkawa Koubunkan, 2013.
Glassman, Hank. *The Face of Jizō: Image and Cult in Medieval Japanese Buddhism.* Honolulu: University of Hawai'i Press, 2012.
Gluck, Carol. "The End of Elsewhere: Writing Modernity Now." *The American Historical Review* 116, no. 3 (2011): 676–87.
Gorai, Shigeru. *Ishi no shūkyō.* Tokyo: Kadokawa shoten, 1988.
Gotō, Takanori. *Chinmoku to bakuhatsu: dokyumento "Minamatabyō jiken" 1873–1995.* Tokyo: Shūeisha, 1995.
Grainger, Brett Malcolm. *Church in the Wild: Evangelicals in Antebellum America.* Cambridge, MA: Harvard University Press, 2019.

Greene, Gayle. "Science with a Skew: The Nuclear Power Industry after Chernobyl and Fukushima." *The Asia-Pacific Journal* 10, issue 1, no. 3 (2011), https://apjjf.org/2012/10/1/Gayle-Greene/3672/article.html

Hagihara, Shūko. "Umiotosareru kotoba, tewatasareteiku kotoba: MInamatabyō jiken to 'Hongan no kai,'" *Shūkyō kenkyū,* 373 (2011): 203–30.

Hanazaki, Kōhei. *"Janaka shaba" no tetsugaku: jendā, esunishiteī, ekologī.* Tokyo: Inpakuto shuppankai, 2002.

Hara, Takeshi. "Intabyū Ogata Masato: 'Bunmei no kakumei' o machinozomu—Hongan towa nani ka." In *Kyoto Kankyōgaku: Shūkyōsei to ekorojī,* edited by Hara Takeshi. Tokyo: Fujiwara shoten, 2013.

Harada, Masazumi. *Minamatabyō.* Tokyo: Iwanami shoten, 1972.

_______. *Yutakasa to kimin tachi: Minamatagaku kotohajime.* Tokyo: Iwanami shoten. 2007.

_______. *Takarago tachi: Taijisei MInamatabyō ni mananda 50nen.* Fukuoka: Gen shobō, 2009.

_______. *Harada Masazumi tsuitoushū: Kono michi o—Minamata kara,* edited by Kumamoto nichinichi shinbun and Kumamoto gakuen daigaku MInamatagaku kenkyū sentā. Kumamoto: Kumamoto nichinichi shimbunsha, 2012.

Harada, Masazumi, and Tajiri Masami. "Shounisei • taijisei Minamatabyō ni kansuru rinshou ekigakuteki kenkyū." *The Study of Social Relations* 14, no. 1 (2009): 1–66.

Harada, Nobuo. *Rekishi no naka no kome to niku: Shokumotsu to ten'no/sabetsu.* Tokyo: Heibonsha, 2013 [2005].

Harootunian, Harry. "Memory, mourning, and national morality: Yasukuni Shrine and the reunion of state and religion in postwar Japan." In *Nation and Religion: Perspectives on Europe and Asia,* edited by Peter Van Der Veer and Harmut Lehmann. Princeton: Princeton University Press, 1999.

Harris, Sheldon H. *Factories of Death: Japanese Biological Warfare, 1932–1945, and the American Cover-up.* London: Routledge, 2002.

Hatakeyama, Shigeatsu. *Mori wa umi no koibito.* Tokyo: Bungei shunjū, 2006.

_______. *Mori wa tetsu de yomigaeru.* Tokyo: Bungei shunjū, 2012.

Higashijima, Dai. *Naze Minamatabyō wa kaiketsu dekinai noka.* Fukuoka: Gen shobō, 2010.

Ikeda, Richiko, and Tanaka Yasuhiro ed. *Jidai o kiku: Okinawa Minamata Yokkaichi Niigata Fukushima.* Tokyo: Serika shobō, 2012.

Ingold, Tim. *Perception of the Environment: Essays on Livelihood, Dwelling and Skill.* London: Routledge, 2000.

Irokawa, Daikichi. *Minamata—Sono sabetsu no fūdo to rekihsi, Shiranui kai ichi chōsadanin no shōgen* (Minamata—The history of its discrimination and climate, a testimony of a member of Shiranui Sea Investigation team). Minamata: Hankōgai Minamata kyoutoukaigi jimukyoku, 1980.

Ishida, Hirofumi. *Minamatabyō to rōdōsha: Chisso Minamata no rōdōsha wa Minamatabyō to dou mukiattanoka.* Kumamoto: Ishida Hirofumi, 2013.

Ishimure, Michiko, and Tsurumi Kazuko. *Kotoba hatsuru tokoro—Tsurumi Kazuko • taiwa mandara Ihimure Michiko no maki.* Tokyo: Fujiwara shoten, 2002.

Ishimure, Michiko. *Paradise in the Sea of Sorrow: Our Minamata Disease.* Translated by Livia Monnet. Ann Arbor, MI: Center for Japanese Studies, University of Michigan, 2003.

Ishimure, Michiko, and Tada Michio. *Kotodama.* Tokyo: Fujiwara shoten. 2008.

———. *Soseishita Tamashii o nosete.* Tokyo: Kawaide shobōshinsha, 2013.

———. *Yoshi no Nagisa: Ishimure Michiko jiden.* Tokyo: Fujiwara shoten, 2014.

———. *Tamashii no hikyō kara.* Tokyo: Asahi shimbunsha, 2018.

Josephson-Storm, Jason Ā. *The Myth of Disenchantment: Magic, Modernity, and the Birth of the Human Sciences.* Chicago: University of Chicago Press, 2017.

Kamanaka, Hitomi. *Hibakusha: Sekai no owari.* 2003.

———. *Rokkashomura Rapusodī.* 2006.

———. *Chiisaki koe no kanon.* 2010.

Kamoi, Yū. *Noguchi Shitagau: Ningen to jigyō.* Tokyo: Tōkōsha, 1943.

Kan, Chae-On. *Chōsen ni okeru Nitchitsu kontserun.* Tokyo: Fuji shuppan, 1986.

Kasuya, Ken'ichi. "Seiji Keizai to Chōsen ni okeru nitchitsu zaibatsu no tenkai" *Chōsenshi kenkyūkai Ronbunshū* 12 (1975): 175–209.

Kawabe, Shigeru. *Uo wa ningen no te dewa tsukurenai: Genpatsu de kurushimu gyomin no tachiba kara.* Tokyo: Jushinsha, 1984.

Kayashima, Hidenobu. "Fusenkō hatsuden kouji to Kōnan koujou no kensetsu." In *Kikigaki Minamata Minshūshi* 5, *Shokuminchi wa tengoku datta.* Edited by Okamoto Tatsuaki and Mitsuzaki Tsuuo. Tokyo: Sōfūkan, 1997 [1990].

Ketain, AnaLouise. "'I'm a Citizen of the Universe': Gloria Anzalúa's Spiritual Activism as Catalyst for Social Change." *Feminist Studies,* 34, no. ½ (2008): 53–69.

Kikuchi, Daisuke. "In First, Government and TEPCO Found Liable for Fukushima Disaster." *The Japan Times,* March 17, 2017. https://www.japantimes.co.jp/news/2017/03/17/national/crime-legal/first-government-tepco-found-liable-fukushima-disaster/

Kimura, Mitsuhiko. "The Economics of Japanese Imperialism in Korea, 1910–1939." *Economic History Review, New Series* 48, no. 3 (August 1995): 555–74.

King, Tiffany Lethabo, Janell Navarro, and Andrea Smith. *Otherwise Worlds: Against Settler Colonialism and Anti-Blackness.* Durham, NC: Duke University Press, 2020.

Klein, Naomi. *Shock Doctrine: The Rise of Disaster Capitalism.* New York: Picador, 2007.

Knecht, Peter. "Rice Representations and Reality." *Asian Folk Religion and Culture* 66 (2007): 5–25.

Kobayashi, Naoki. "*Minamata no gensetsu to hyōshō.* Tokyo: Fujiwara shoten, 2007.

Kobayashi, Toshiyuki. "Nihonjin no shūkyōteki ishiki ya dōdō wa dou kawattaka—ISSP Kokusai hikaku chōsa 'Shūkyō' Nihon no kekka kara." *Hōsō kenkyū to chōsa* 69, no. 4 (2019): 52–72.

Koga, Tōru. *Risei no bōryoku: Nihonshakai no byōrigaku.* Tokyo: Seitousha, 2014.

Kojima, Takeshi. *Higashi ajia kaiiki ni kogidasu.* Tokyo: Tokyo daigaku shuppankai, 2013.

Komatsu, Hiroshi. *Shin no bunmei wa hito o korosazu: Tanaka Shouzou no kotoba ni manabu asu no nihon.* Tokyo: Shōgakkan, 2011.

Komatsubara, Orika. "'Kougai mondai' kara 'kankyō mondai' e: Minamata chiiki ni okeru 'Shiranui kai sōgō gakujutsu chōsadan' no katsudou o tegakari ni" *Gendai seimei tetsuaku kenkyū* 7 (March 2018): 74–106.

_______. "'Higaisha no jōnen' kara 'higaisha no hyōgen' e: Minamatabyō 'hitokabu undō' (1970) ni okeru higaisha ・kagaisha taiwa o kentou suru" *Gendai seimei tetsugaku kenkyū.* 8 (March 2019): 57–129.

Koskenniemi, Martti. *The Gentle Civilizer of Nations: The Rise and Fall of International Law 1870–1960.* New York: Cambridge University Press, 2001.

Krämer, Hans Martin. "'Not Befitting Our Divine Country': Eating Meat in Japanese Discourses of Self and Other from the Seventeenth Century to the Present" *Food and Foodways* 16 (2008): 33–62.

Kripal, Jeffrey J. *Authors of the Impossible: the Paranormal and the Sacred.* Chicago: University of Chicago Press, 2010.

Kurahashi, Yoko. "Creating a Tapestry of Voice and Silence in Michiko Ishimure's 'Kugai jōdo' (Paradise in the Sea of Sorrow)." *Journal of Narrative Theory* 33, no. 3 (2003): 315–34.

Kurihara, Akira. *Shōgen Minamatabyō.* Tokyo: Iwanami shoten, 2000.

Kurihara, Akira and Fujiwara Tatsushi. "Keshō no oto o kiku" *Gendai shisō,* 46, no. 7 (2018).

LaFleur, William R. *Liquid Life: Abortion and Buddhism in Japan.* Princeton: Princeton University Press, 1994.

Lamarre, Thomas. *The Anime Ecology: A Genealogy of Television, Animation, and Game Media.* Minneapolis, MN: University of Minnesota Press, 2018.

Levinas, Emmanuel. *Totality and Infinity: An Essay on Exteriority.* Pittsburgh, PA: Duquesne University Press, 1969.

Levinas, Emmanuel. *Otherwise than Being of Beyond Essence.* Translated by Alphonso Lingis. Norwell, MA: Kluwer Academic Publishers, 1991.

Lewis, Thomas A. *Why Philosophy Matters for the Study of Religion & Vice Versa.* New York: Oxford University Press, 2015.

Mahmood, Saba. "Religious Reason and Secular Affect: An Incommensurable Divide?" In *Is Critique Secular? Blasphemy, Injury, and Free Speech.* Contributed by Talal Asad, Wendy Brown, Judith Butler, and Saba Mahmood. Berkeley, CA: University of California Press, 2009.

Marran, Christine L. *Ecology without Culture: Aesthetics for a Toxic World.* Minneapolis, MN: University of Minnesota Press, 2017.

Maruyama, Sadami, Taguchi Hiroaki, and Tanaka Yūji, ed. *Minamata kara no souzouryoku: Toitsuzukeru Minamatabyō.* Kumamoto: Sōryū shuppan, 2005.

Masuda, Shōzō. *Zeami no sekai.* Tokyo: Shūeisha, 2007.

Masuo, Shin'ichirō, and Joseph P. Elacqua. "Chinese Religion and the Formation of Onmyōdō." *Japanese Journal of Religion Studies* 40, no. 1 (2013): 19–43.

Masuzawa, Tomoko. *The Invention of World Religions, or, How European Universalism Was Preserved in the Language of Pluralism.* Chicago: University of Chicago Press, 2005.

Matsunaga, Daigan, and Alicia Matsunaga. "The Concept of Upāya in Mahāyāna Buddhist Philosophy." *Japanese Journal of Religious Studies* 1, no. 1 (1974): 51–72.

Matsuya, Rie. "Kūkan no keiken to shite no fuukei: Yi-Fu Tuan kara Ishimure Michiko e" *Kokusai Bunkagaku Kenkyū* 38 (2012): 1–21.

McGrath, Alister. *The Reenchantment of Nature: The Denial of Religion and the Ecological Crisis.* New York: Doubleday, 2002.

McGraw, Peter, and Jowl Warner, "The Danish Cartoon Crisis of 2005 and 2006: 10 Things You Didn't Know About the Original Muhammad Controversy." *Huffington Post,* September 24, 2012, https://www.huffpost.com/entry/muhammad-cartoons_b_1907545?guccounter=1&guce_referrer=aHR0cHM6Ly93d3cuZ29vZ2xlLmNvbS8&guce_referrer_sig=AQAAAKrDzX2ApKgROrZIrwYsdeM7dD-Drjt5hnrHwG4f-6_7zZGW-RH-HWtEhCZrvUwSMw5d9Tf7cHt9IM4ypubyKnhGV-EJkx6lI680AEGSL51dxVoPgm-Se60cKwgV-aJ07djohGGntwnBLgFMTF8H5Lp_XQxWe7w6TvUHGLQsKIVO

Melzer, Juergen P. "Review: Constructing East Asia: Technology, Ideology, and Empire in Japan's Wartime Era, 1931–1945." *Japan Review* 27 (2014): 243–45.

Miller, Alan L. "Spiritual Accomplishment by Misdirection: Some 'Upāya' Folktales from East Asia." *History of Religions* 40, no. 1 (2000): 82–108.

Miller, Ian Jared, Julia Adeney Thomas, and Brett L. Walker, ed. *Japan at Nature's Edge: The Environmental Context of a Global Power.* Honolulu: University of Hawai'i Press, 2013.

Mine, Takeshi. "'Manshū' kagaku kougyou no kaihatsu to shin Chūgoku e no keishou." *Ajia kenkyū* 52, no. 1 (2006): 19–43.

Miyamoto, Tsuneichi. *Umi ni ikiru hitobito.* Tokyo: Kawaide shobō shinsha. 2015.

Mizutamari, Mayumi. "Ishimure Michiko to 'rumin.'" *Gendai shisō* 46, no. 7 (2018).

Molony, Barbara. *Technology and Investment: The Prewar Japanese Chemical Industry.* Cambridge: Harvard University Press, 1990.

Monnet, Livia. "'Another World in This World': Slow violence, Environmental Time, and the Decolonial Imagination in Ishimure Michiko's *Villages of the Gods.*" In *Ishimure Michiko's Writing in Ecocritical Perspective: Between Sea and Sky,* edited by Bruce Allen and Yuki Masami. Lanham, MD: Lexington Books, 2015.

Moore, Aaron Stephen. *Constructing East Asia: Technology, Ideology, and Empire in Japan's Wartime Era, 1931–1945.* Stanford: Stanford University Press, 2013.

Morishita, Naoki. "Minamatabyō shi ni okeru 'Shiranui kai sōgō gakujutsu chōsadan' no ichi—jinbun shakaikagaku kenkyū no 'kyōdō koui' ni tsuite" in *Seizongaku kenkyū sentā hōkoku,* "Kotonari" no rikigaku—mainoritī o meguru kenkyū to houhou no jissenteki kadai, edited by Yamamoto Takanori and Takahashi Shin'ichi 14 (2010): 319–348.

Moro-Sanchez, Milla Micka. "Jizō, Healing Rituals, and Women in Japan." *Japanese Journal of Religious Studies* 43, no. 2 (2016): 307–31.

Morton, Timothy. *Hyperobjects: Philosophy and Ecology after the End of the World.* Minneapolis, MN: University of Minnesota Press, 2013.

Mosse, George L. *Fallen Soldiers: Reshaping the Memory of the World Wars.* New York: Oxford University Press, 1991.

Murakami, Haruki. *Shokugyō to shite no shōsetsuka*. Tokyo: Sinchōsha, 2015.

Nakamura, Ikuo. *Saishi to kugi: Nihonjin no shizenkan dōbutsukan*. Kyoto: Hōzōkan, 2001.

Nakazawa, Shin'ichi. *Wakusei no fūkei: Nakazawa Shin'ichi taidanshū*. Tokyo: Seidosha, 2014.

Naumann, Nelly. "Whale and Fish Cult in Japan: A Basic Feature of Ebisu Worship." *Asian Folklore Studies* 33, no. 1 (1974): 1–15.

Nihon keieishi kenkyūsho. *Fūsetsu no hyakunen: Chisso kabushikigaisha shi*. Tokyo: Chisso kabushikigaisha, 2011.

Nixon, Rob. 2011. *Slow Violence and the Environmentalism of the Poor*. Cambridge, MA. Harvard University Press.

Odagiri, Hiroyuki, and Gotō Akira. *Technology and Industrial Development in Japan: Building Capabilities by Learning, Innovation and Public Policy*. Oxford: Clarendon Press, 1996.

Ogata, Masato. *Tokoy no fune o kogite*. Yokohama: Seori shobō, 1996.

———. *Rowing the Eternal Sea: The Story of a Minamata Fisherman*. Interview by Oiwa Keibo. Translated by Karen Collingan-Taylor. Lanham, MD: Rowman & Littlefield, 2001.

———. *Chisso wa watashi de atta*. Fukuoka: Ashi shobō, 2001.

Oishi, Yutaka. "Sengo Nihon no shakaiundō ni okeru Chisso rōdōundō no ichizuke—mou hitotsu no Minamata." *Ohara shakai mondai kenkyūsho zasshi* 630 (2011): 14–28.

Okamoto, Tatsuaki. *Minamatabyō no minshūshi*, vol. 1 *Mae no jidai—butai to shite no mittsu no mura to Minamata wan*. Tokyo: Nihon hyōronsh, 2015.

Onishi, Norimatsu, and Martin Fackler. "Japan Held Nuclear Data, Leaving Evacuees in Peril." *The New York Times*, August 8, 2011. https://www.nytimes.com/2011/08/09/world/asia/09japan.html

Oshio, Takeshi. "Reimeiki kābaido bijinesu no keifu to Noguchi Jun—Sankyozawa Kābaido seizōsho kara Nihon Chisso Hiryō ni itaru michisuji." *The papers and proceedings of economics* 153 (2017): 133–54.

Ōuchi, Fumi. "Musical Instruments for the Sea-God Ebisu: The Mythological System of Miho Shrine and Its Performative Power." In *The Sea and the Sacred in Japan: Aspects of Maritime Religion,* edited by Fabio Rambelli. London: Bloomsbury, 2018.

Oyabu, Junko. "Fukushima genpatsujiko kara 8nenme 'hinansha o shiensuru hinansha' wa nani o omou." *Diamond online,* August 24, 2018. https://diamond.jp/articles/-/178130

Park, Soon Won. "The First Generation of Korean Skilled Workers: the Onoda Cement Sŭunghori Factory." *The Journal of Korean Studies* 7 (1990): 55–96.

Rambelli, Fabio. "General Introduction: The Sea in the History of Japanese Religions." In *The Sea and the Sacred in Japan: Aspects of Maritime Religion,* edited by Fabio Rambelli. London: Bloomsbury, 2018.

_______. "Sea Theologies: Elements for a Conceptualization of Maritime Religiosity in Japan" In *The Sea and the Sacred in Japan: Aspects of Maritime Religion,* edited by Fabio Rambelli. London: Bloomsbury, 2018.

Rasch, William. "Enlightenment as Religion." *New German Critique* 36, no. 3 (2009): 109–31.
Rots, Aike P. "Sacred Forests, Sacred Nation: The Shinto Environmentalist Paradigm and the Rediscovery of *Chinju no Mori*." *Japanese Journal of Religious Studies* 42, no. 2 (2015): 205–33.
Saishu, Satoru. *Ashita mo mata kyou no gotoku* (Tomorrow is like today). Tokyo: Dōbutsusha, 1988.
Sakurada, Katsunori. *Umi no shūkyō*. Kyoto: Tankōsha, 1970.
Sakurai Eiji. *Zouyo no erkishigaku: Girei to Keizai no aida*. Tokyo: Chūō kōron shinsha, 2011.
Shibusawa, Keizō. "Engishiki nai suisan shinsen ni kansuru kousatsu jakkan." In *Shibusawa Keizō chosakushū* 1 (1993).
Shimura, Fukumi, and Ishimure Michiko. *Yuigon: taidan to oufukushokan*. Tokyo: Chikuma shobō, 2014.
Shinmoto, Masafumi. "Minamatabyō jiken ni okeru 'daisansha kikan' no mondai." *Kyushu Kyōritsu Daigaku Keizaigakubu Kiyō* 114 (2008): 1–20.
Shiota, Takeshi. *Minamata na hito—Minamatabyō o shien shita hitobito no kiseki*. Tokyo: Miraisha. 2013.
Sontag, Susan. *Illness as Metaphor and AIDS and Its Metaphors*. New York: Picado, 1989 [1988].
Stolz, Robert. *Bad Water: Nature, Pollution, and Politics in Japan, 1870–1950*. Durham, NC: Duke University Press, 2014.
Strange, Susan. *Casino Capitalism*. Manchester: Manchester University Press, 1997.
Sugisawa, Haruko. "Noh no monogurui ni tsuite no kenkyū." *Yūgō bunka kenkyū* 7 (2006): 66–81.
Sunada, Akira. *Umi yo haha yo kodomora yo: Yumekanjin no sekai*. Tokyo: Jushinsha, 1983.
Sze, Julie. "From Environmental Justice Literature to the Literature of Environmental Justice." In *The Environmental Justice Reader*, edited by Joni Adamson, Mei Mei Evans, and Rachel Stein, 163–180. Tucson: University of Arizona Press, 2002.
Takahashi, Shin'ichi, and Wakabayashi Yoshikazu. "Tankou roudousha no idou to kyū santanchi no shakai hendou" (Social Change and Labor Mobility in the Coal Industry). *Shakaigaku kenkyūsho kiyou* 11 (1990): 45–77.
Takamine, Takeshi. *Minamatabyō o shitte imasuka*. Tokyo: Iwanami shoten, 2016.
Tanaka, Satoshi. *Kenkou hō to iyashi no shakaishi*. Tokyo: Seikyūsha, 2006.
———. *Denki wa dare no monoka*. Tokyo: Shōbunsha, 2015.
Tani, Ken'ichi. *1961nen: Yoru ni noboru taiyō*, 2018.
Tanno, Haruka. "Yanagida Kōichi to 'Minamatabyō o tsutaeru' katsudō: Shisui no kihon kōzō o chūshin ni." *Kankyōkyōiku* 25, no. 1 (2015): 48–59.
Thomas, Julia Adeney. *Reconfiguring Modernity: Concepts of Nature in Japanese Political Ideology*. Berkeley: University of California Press, 2002.
Thornber, Karen. "Ishimure Michiko and Global Ecocriticism" *The Asia-Pacific Journal* 14, issue 13, no. 6 (2016). https://apjjf.org/2016/13/Thornber.html
Tian, Min. "Chinese Nuo and Japanese Noh: Nuo's Role in the Origination and formation of Noh." *Comparative Drama* 37, no. ¾ (2003–2004): 343–60.

Togashi, Sadao. *Minamatabyō jiken to hou.* Fukuoka: Sekifūsha, 1995.

Tōyō Bōseki. *Tōyō Bōseki 70-nen shi.* Osaka: Tōyō Bōseki, 1953.

Toyosato, Mayumi. "Mapping Nonmodernity: Home and the World in Ishimure Michiko's *Kugai jōdo.*" In *Ishimure Michiko's Writing in Ecocritical Perspective: Between Sea and Sky,* edited by Bruce Allen and Yuki Masami. Lanham, MD: Lexington Books, 2016.

Tsuchiya, Keiichirō. *Noh: Dorama ga tachiawarareru toki.* Tokyo: Kadokawa, 2014.

Tsujihara, Makihiko. "Chōsen Chisso Hiryō no Kōnan chiku shatakugai nit suite—Noguchi kenkyusho shozou shiryou o mochiite—" (Restoration of the company town plan constructed by the Chosen Chisso Niryo Hungnam Factory—Using materials owned by the Noguchi Institute). *Nihon kenchiku gakkai keikaku kei ronbunshū* 77, no. 671 (January 2012): 135–42.

Tweed, Thomas A. *Crossing and Dwelling: A Theory of Religion.* Cambridge: Harvard University Press, 2006.

Uchiyama, Takashi. *Kyōdōtai no kisoriron—Shizen to ningen no kisō kara* (The Basic Logic of a Community—From the Foundation of Nature and Humans). Tokyo: Nōson gyoson bunka kyōkai, 2010.

Walker, Brett L. *Toxic Archipelago: A History of Industrial Disease in Japan.* Seattle: University of Washington Press, 2011.

Watanabe, Kyōji. *Mou hitotsu no konoyo: Ishimure Michiko no uchū.* Fukuoka: Gen shobō, 2013.

Watanabe, Shin'ichi, and Seki Reiko. "'Dai-san Minamatabyō' mondai no genzaiteki isou I: 'Dai-san Minamatabyō' to suigin panikku." *Oitakenritsu geijutsubunka tankidaigaku kenkyū kiyō 33* (1995): 47–66.

Weber, Max. "Science as a Vocation." *Daedalus* 87, no. 1 (1958): 111–134.

White, Brent T. "Reexamining Separation: The Construction of Separation of Religion and State in Post-War Japan." *Pacific Basin Law Journal* 22, no. 1 (2004): 29–88.

White, Stephen K. "As the World Turns: Ontology and Politics in Judith Butler." *Polity* 32, no. 2 (1999): 155–77.

———. "Weak Ontology: Genealogy and Critical Issues." *Hedgehog Review* 7, no. 2 (2005). https://hedgehogreview.com/issues/weak-ontologies/articles/weak-ontology-genealogy-and-critical-issues

Wyschogrod, Edith. *Saints and Postmodernism: Revisioning Moral Philosophy.* Chicago: University of Chicago Press, 1990.

Yahagi, Tadashi. "Chisso shi 1970–75, I." *Urawa Ronsō* 33 (2004): 43–80.

Yamaguchi, Osamu. *Amakusa: Hito to rekishi.* Kyoto: Tankōshinsha [Tankōsha], 1966.

Yamashita, Shun'ichi. "Japan Admits 3 Nuclear Meltodowns, More Radiaiton Leaked into Sea; U.S. Nuclear Waste Poses Deadly Risks." *Democracy Now*, June 10, 2011. https://www.democracynow.org/2011/6/10/as_japan_nuclear_crisis_worsens_citizen

Yasumuro, Satoru. "'Hyakushō ryōshi' to 'Ryōshi hyakushō': Umitsuki no mura no seigyō fukugou to suiden inasaku." *Kokuritsu rekishi minzoku hakubutsukan kenkyū hōkoku,* 162 (2011): 323–43.

Yonemoto, Kōji. *Hyouden Ishimure Michiko: Nagisa ni tatsu hito.* Tokyo: Shinchōsha, 2017.

Yoneyama, Shoko. "Life-world: Beyond Fukushima and Minamata." *Japan focus: Asia-Pacific Journal* 10, issue 42, no. 2 (2012). https://apjjf.org/2012/10/42/Shoko-YONEYAMA/3845/article.html

———. *Animism in Contemporary Japan: Voices for the Anthropocene from Post-Fukushima Japan.* New York: Routledge, 2019.

Yoshikawa, Muneaki. *Ganseki o shinkō shite ita Nihonjin: Ishigami, iwakura, iwa-saku, kigan, kyoseki to yobareru mono no kenkyū.* Osaka: Yū taimu shuppan, 2011.

Yoshimi, Shunya. *"Koe" no shihonshugi.* Tokyo: Kōdansha, 1995.

Žižek, Slavoj. *The Parallax View.* Cambridge: MIT Press, 2006.

_______. "Ecology." *Examined Life: Excursions with Contemporary Thinkers,* edited by Astra Taylor. New York: The New Press, 2009.

_______. "Reborn from the Earth Scarred by Modernity: Minamata Disease and the Miracle of the Human Desire to Live." Translated by Michael Bourdaghs. *Asia-Pacific Journal* 6, issue 4, no. 0 (2008).

Index

About the Author

Yuki Miyamoto is associate professor at DePaul University. Since having earned her PhD from the University of Chicago (ethics; Divinity School), her work centers around the nuclear discourse—a monograph, *Beyond the Mushroom Cloud: Commemoration, Religion, and Responsibility after Hiroshima* (2011), and several articles (ex. "In the Light of Hiroshima: Banalizing Violence and Normalizing Experiences of the Atomic Bombing," "Gendered Bodies in *Tokusatsu*: Reproduction and Representation of the Atomic Bomb Victims," etc.). After 2011's Fukushima nuclear accident, she has observed uncanny commonalities between nuclear disasters and environmental destructions, such as methylmercury poisoning observed in Minamata.

www.ingramcontent.com/pod-product-compliance
Ingram Content Group UK Ltd.
Pitfield, Milton Keynes, MK11 3LW, UK
UKHW020841290926
15470UKWH00004B/1490

9 781793 643605